I0560536

CAN YOU TRUST YOUR DENTIST?

What You Need to Know Before Your Next Dental Appointment

MARK MORGAN, DDS, MBA

Copyright ©

Publication year 2024

Owner: Active Science Press LLC

Mark R. Morgan, author

Mark R. Morgan, II, editor

All rights reserved. This book or any part thereof may not be reproduced, used for artificial intelligence in any fashion, stored in a retrieval system, or transmitted in any form or by any means, electronic, mechanical, photocopying, or otherwise, without prior written permission of the publisher.

Ordering information: Paperback copies are available directly from Active Science Press LLC.

Edition One

ISBN: 979-8-9874251-2-1 Paperback

ISBN: 979-8-9874251-0-7 EPUB

ISBN: 979-8-9874251-3-8 Kindle

Library of Congress Control Number 2023924241

Cover and interior book design by Damonza.

Illustrations by Ajay Joshi

I dedicate this book to my readers interested in taking an active role in protecting their dental health.

Table of Contents

Illustrations

Acknowledgments

I want to thank my colleagues, wife, and children for their considerable help and patience throughout the creation of this book.

Introduction

We never learn the terminology or what is important about oral health in elementary school, high school, or college. Even medical doctors only receive a few hours of education about dentistry.

Unbiased sources comparing the benefits and risks of different dental treatments are nearly impossible to find. I wrote this book to provide an easy-to-understand reference for evaluating your dental treatment options.

My experience in dentistry is extensive and varied. I performed nearly 10,000 surgeries as a periodontist and general dentist. I worked in both private practice and for multi-location corporate dental offices. I ran a large practice and employed other dentists. I spent nearly a decade teaching dental students and dental hygiene students. I have testified as an expert witness in the courtroom. I worked as a volunteer dentist at a free clinic in Southern California. I spent a summer working as a volunteer for migrant farm workers in mobile clinic buses. I was a paid consultant, and my office was a clinical trial site, for the evaluation of local antibiotic placement products and dental bone graft materials.

What I am stating in this book is my opinion.

This book will help you understand what to expect with specific treatments and avoid the risks associated with some costly popular procedures. If something went wrong with your dental treatment, this book describes the likely reasons for the failed therapy. You will learn what is most important to do in order to keep your teeth for a lifetime. You will know how to avoid procedures that are likely to create complications and repeated dental visits. I want to help everyone be more educated about their teeth and dentistry.

This book also suggests ways to identify quality dentists and avoid bad dentists and the disappointing treatments they may recommend.

You will benefit from reading this book before you receive an informed consent disclosure (and treatment). While disclosures are supposed to educate you about risks, benefits, and alternatives, they are generally not as complete or easy to understand as what is disclosed in this book. You usually are provided with the form immediately before the treatment when you might be experiencing nervousness and time pressure to move forward with the appointment. This information is sometimes provided to you after you have been given a sedative (or self-sedated). Long-term risks and results are rarely discussed fully. The following chapters will also provide you with an understanding of the rarely discussed negative aspects about each dental treatment.

Each chapter is stand-alone, so you can go to the dental topic of your choice and quickly gain a good understanding of such issues as these:

- *Gum disease*. Understanding and controlling gum disease can prevent the main cause of tooth loss by adults. Failure to understand gum disease and just delegating this aspect to your dentist and hygienist can result in serious tooth loss.

- *Dental implants.* Many readers will be considering dental implants. My background as a periodontist and implantologist gives me the experience to advise you about the most expensive dental decision you may face. I have written four extensive chapters on dental implants and both the joys and the problems experienced by patients once dental implants are placed.

- *Trauma.* The chapter on trauma provides you with the scientific consensus on recommended treatment after various types of trauma to teeth.

- *Dentures.* If you have problems with dentures, I have itemized solutions for every problem I have ever seen or heard about.

- *Sleep Apnea.* A comprehensive chapter is dedicated to explaining the risks and benefits of all the various options used by physicians and dentists for treating obstructive sleep apnea.

- *Choosing a good dentist.* Most importantly, perhaps, is chapter nineteen on how to choose a good dentist.

The health of your mouth and teeth is one of the most important contributors to your overall health. Having good dental health influences your appearance and can help you socially and professionally. Your good dental health further contributes to your ability to get hired and stay employed. Research shows that if you feel comfortable talking and smiling you exude more confidence, work comfortably in groups, do better at sales, and get promoted.

It is often easy to determine that you need dental treatment. The difficulty comes when you must choose from alternative treatment choices presented by your dentist. An ideal treatment choice for one person may be the worst choice for another. Each treatment choice comes with associated risks and expected results. This book will help you make the right choice for your unique medical, financial, and family situation. This book cannot substitute, however, for obtaining a diagnosis from a dentist or physician who knows the details of your oral health history.

This material is for informational purposes only and is not a substitute for medical or dental advice. I hope it will make you a more informed person, so that you will never regret your dental treatment choices.

One

Gum Disease

Gum disease is a main reason why adults lose their teeth. This is because people do not seek treatment for gum disease soon enough since it does not hurt until advanced stages. Additionally, many dentists fail to recognize or properly treat gum disease until it is too late. Let's examine how and why gum disease (also called periodontal disease or periodontitis) develops, why it is missed in early stages, and the treatment options.

From the Dawning to the Daunting

From the moment that our teeth erupt through the gums into our mouths, we have a normal and healthy set of bacteria growing on the visible areas of our teeth and under the gumline. This initial bacterial colony exists in harmony with our immune system and is compatible with good health. There are a few stages in the progression of gum disease that need to be understood. These stages are discussed in the next sections of this chapter.

Initial colonization

When new bacteria get into our mouths, the bacteria float around in saliva until they randomly come across a spot where they can exist. This place is where the bacteria have the right amount of nutrients and something they can stick to. If they stick to a spot on your tongue or inner cheek they will come off in a few days when your skin cells shed normally. Therefore, the main place where they can live for more than a few days is on the hard surfaces of the teeth.

We are initially exposed to these bacteria from food or people's saliva when we are infants. This exposure to new bacteria continues throughout our lives.

Plaque (biofilm)

When bacteria find a spot they like, they make a sugary glue that allows them to stay stuck to that surface. This glue, plus the bacteria, is called *plaque* or *biofilm*. The bacteria then start to divide and grow into a bigger colony. If they are near the gumline, the bacteria divide and push their progeny under the gums. The bacteria that are under the gums tend to grow quickly and proliferate because they are not knocked loose by hard food or reached by toothbrush bristles.

Bacteria are continually dividing, but each individual bacterium lives only a couple of days. When bacteria in dental plaque die, salt in the saliva deposits into the dead cell bodies. When this happens to a lot of adjacent bacteria, a structure develops that is like a coral reef in the ocean.

Calculus

When bacterial plaque hardens, the hard substance is called *calculus* (tartar). The attachment of calculus to a tooth is particularly strong. The bond to the tooth gets stronger as it ages making the calculus tougher and harder to remove. When bacteria are newly stuck to the teeth and are making their glue attachment, they can be removed with toothbrush bristles or floss. Once the bacteria die and start to harden into calculus, the attachment to the tooth is too strong to be removed by toothbrush bristles, floss, or water-pulsing devices. Sequential colonies of bacteria can live for decades in the structure of this coral-like calculus. The bacterial colonies get bigger and destroy the gum attachment to the tooth, allowing for deeper penetration below the gumline. Because this process is slow, you do not usually feel any pain or discomfort. The only hint you have of disease progression is bleeding gums when toothbrushing. Bleeding gums almost always indicate at least early gum disease is present.

Gingivitis

Gingivitis is not a true disease, but a gingival inflammation. This inflammation is similar to redness next to a pimple or a splinter. The inflammation is caused by the presence of microorganisms such as bacteria accumulating next to the gum tissue. We treat gingivitis by removing bacteria with brushing and flossing and a general cleaning in a dental office. Bone loss is not seen in gingivitis.

Periodontitis (periodontal disease)

Periodontitis is the disease that occurs when the gum tissue and bone holding your teeth are destroyed due to the presence of bacteria and other microorganisms. The main cause of adult tooth loss is this localized, usually painless, destruction of your gum and bone tissue. This disease can be caused by numerous species of bacteria that grow into colonies down under the gums. The bacteria slide into the same space between your gums and teeth where you can get popcorn husks stuck when you eat popcorn. Your immune system's reaction to the bacteria causes much of the bone destruction. This is because your body releases proteins, called cytokines, which create an inflammatory response that mobilizes white blood cells to attack the bacteria. The inflammatory response by your body kills the bacteria. This attack on the bacteria is a bit sloppy and also destroys the bone and gums in the area around the bacteria. This inflammatory response also causes the tissues to bleed easily.

Bacteria that live above the gumline use oxygen and are called aerobic bacteria. They produce the odorless gas carbon dioxide from the food they digest. The most destructive bacterial species are called anaerobic bacteria; they cannot tolerate oxygen and hide in deep unoxygenated areas in your mouth. The most common space for these bacteria to live are deep in the spaces under your gums next to the roots of the teeth. The anaerobic bacteria are particularly prevalent when the space gets to be 5 mm or deeper where there is less oxygen from air in your mouth.

These anaerobic bacteria produce an odor that smells like sulfur or rotten eggs. People with a large amount of gum disease have a buildup of anaerobic bacteria in their mouths and permanently bad breath.

The deep spaces next to the teeth are called periodontal pockets. As the pockets get deeper, there is room for larger colonies of destructive anaerobic bacteria. In addition, more aggressive types of bacterial species can exist as the pocket gets deeper and more devoid of oxygen. These bacteria and the inflammatory response destroys the bone that holds the teeth. Eventually these spaces deep in the pocket can abscess and a large amount of bone is suddenly lost.

Once the pocket depth is greater than around 8 mm and bleeds easily, the risk of losing the tooth becomes serious unless treated right away. Delaying immediate periodontal treatment when a pocket reaches 8 mm means risking the loss of that tooth and possibly other adjacent teeth. An 8 mm pocket can have an episode of rapid bone loss at any time. In addition, aggressive bacterial species growing in this oxygen-depleted deep pocket can leak out and spread to other teeth.

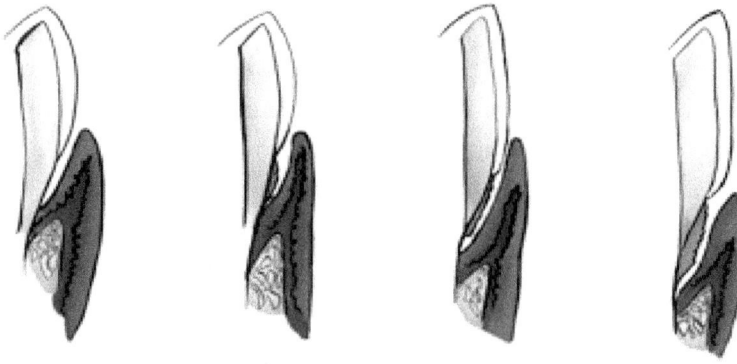

Figure 1.1. Progression of gum disease.

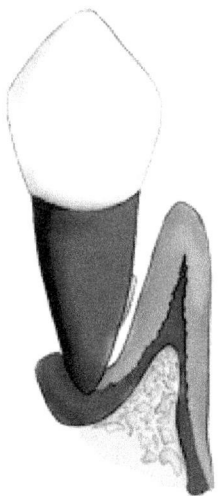

*Figure 1.2. Periodontal disease has destroyed all
gum and bone support on this tooth.*

Treatment

Despite our best efforts at brushing, flossing, and using water-pulsing devices, we can never perfectly clean our teeth due to curves in the tooth shapes and pockets full of bacteria under the gumline. We are absolutely reliant on dentists and dental hygienists to remove bacteria we miss. These professional cleanings prevent bacteria from growing into large colonies that start destroying the gum tissue and bone supporting our teeth. These careful 360-degree efforts to clean around the tooth both above and below the gumline are called scaling and root planing. If the scaling and root planing with curettes and ultrasonic scalers does not control the disease, periodontal surgery is the next stage in treatment.

Scaling and root planing

Scaling is the removal of visible bacteria and calculus above the gumline and root planing is the removal of bacteria and calculus below the gumline. Reducing periodontal pockets to a cleansable 5 mm or less is a main objective of root planing and periodontal surgery. Dental hygienists, dentists, and periodontists find 5 mm or less is a much easier depth to clean. Deeper than 5 mm becomes a daunting and difficult task to clean because the roots do not have uniform shapes below the gumline and the areas cannot be easily visualized. Root planing and periodontal surgery to clean out these deep pockets and keep your teeth are the next two important topics.

Root planing is usually performed as the initial attempt to control periodontal disease. Often you see the dentist for maintenance cleanings every three months once this disease has been detected and root planing has been completed. If the disease stays under control and the pockets are not bleeding upon probing, you may possibly move to a four month or longer cleaning interval. Root planing is often repeated every two years or as needed.

Root planing involves sliding dental instruments to the bottom of the space under the gums to clean the bacteria off the root surface in the areas where the bone and soft gum tissue attachment to the tooth has been destroyed. Root planing usually is tried before surgery.

The objective of root planing is to reduce periodontal infection and shrink up the periodontal pockets so the hygienist and dentist can reach and clean all the bacteria off the teeth more easily at future appointments. Good root planing can often eliminate or reduce the need for more aggressive treatment like periodontal surgery.

Root planing can reduce periodontal pocket depth in three ways.

- Removal of the bacteria with root planing reduces inflammation and brings down the amount of white blood cells and serum leaking from adjacent capillaries into the gum tissue. This results in less puffiness of the gums and the gum tissue shrinks and leaves a shallower periodontal pocket.

- Skin tissue lining the deepest of the periodontal pockets can reattach to the cleaned root surface.

- When the bacteria are removed by root planing, your body quits sending white blood cells to mobilize and wiggle through the tissue lining the bottom of the pocket. This allows the gum tissue cells to reattach tightly to each other since white blood cells are no longer in the way. Once the gum cells grab back onto one another, the tissue is no longer weak and porous. This tightened cuff of tissue at the base of the periodontal pocket results in reduced pocket depth.

If the root planing reduces the pocket depth to less than 5 mm, with good home care you can often return to less frequent professional cleanings.

Root planing is a necessary procedure to control existing periodontal disease. However, like all medical therapies, there are positive and negative aspects of root planing that you should anticipate.

The positive aspects of root planing

The positive aspects of root planing include two major benefits: controlling periodontal disease so you can keep your teeth and eliminating or reducing the need for periodontal surgery.

The negative aspects of root planing

The negative aspects of root planing that you should be aware of include the following:

Discomfort and occasional bleeding after the procedure.

Sometimes a weak filling can be dislodged from the tooth during scaling and root planing because it is difficult to determine if a bump on the tooth below the gums is an edge of a filling or bacteria-laden calculus that needs to be removed.

More root and larger spaces between the teeth can be exposed. The triangular bumps of gum between the teeth are called papillae. When bacteria are present, the papillae can get red and puffy and hide the underlying tissue destruction of the attachment of the bone to the roots. Sometimes the root is exposed when you remove the bacteria and the gums shrink back down to health. If some of the gum and bone tissue has been destroyed by the infection, the gums shrink to a new level. When this happens, the tips of the papilla can shrink and leave a tiny triangular space between the teeth. This can be visually bothersome, but is actually much healthier since it means the pocket depth has decreased and fewer bad bacteria can live there.

Increased root exposure can temporarily lead to more root temperature sensitivity. Keeping your teeth exceptionally clean allows fluoride and ingredients of desensitizing toothpastes to soak into your roots and block the nerves from feeling this sensitivity.

Infection in the gums causes the tissues to have more acid present and acid makes nerves more sensitive. This sensitivity means good root planing usually requires a local anesthetic to be performed comfortably.

Improperly or poorly done root planing

During root planing, the removal of deep bacteria and calculus must be done as carefully and completely as possible. Many differently shaped instruments for the different shapes and sides of the teeth are usually needed to do a good job. Since the bacteria and calculus are below the gums and not visible, the tooth-by-tooth detection and removal of the bacteria requires tactile skill and lots of time to do well. It would be similar to trying to perfectly scrape all barnacles off the hull of a ship while being blindfolded.

Not having root planing performed when needed, or having it done rapidly and poorly, will leave toxic bacterial accumulations under the gums. If root planing is done poorly, the obvious visible bacteria and calculus above the gums or slightly below the gums are removed, but the deeper areas are not reached. This allows the visible areas of the gums to heal and tighten against the tooth, leaving the deeper areas to fester. In fact, cleaning only the bacterial accumulations that are easy to see and reach without cleaning out the deeper areas of infection in the periodontal pockets causes many serious problems.

Only cleaning the visible surface of the teeth and most shallow areas causes the visible tissues to look healthier and occasionally quit bleeding. The patient, dentist, and dental hygienist see a healthier surface and can fail to notice the progression of the bone loss that is going on down deep. (The same problem can occur with rinsing with anti-bacterial mouth rinses: they only reach the surface and upper two or three millimeters of bacteria under the gums and the deep areas are still infected, but the surface looks better.)

Healing and tightening of only the gums near the surface make it harder to slide the cleaning instruments down deep to clean out the infection at the next dental visit. The bacteria that cause the most rapid bone loss cannot tolerate oxygen and do best in an oxygen-free environment. If the surface gums are tighter around the tooth, the deeper areas are more perfectly devoid of oxygen and disease progresses faster.

All these issues will lead to more rapid periodontitis, which is the main reason adults lose their teeth.

Why is inadequate root planing common?

Root planing —done properly and thoroughly—is a powerful weapon to help patients stave off gum disease and keep their teeth over a lifetime. Unfortunately, inadequate root planing is extremely common. In my experience, these eight factors are the most significant reasons why:

1. It is extremely difficult to do excellent root planing beyond 5 millimeters under the gumline. No root planing or poor root planing allows periodontal disease to progress with resultant tooth loss and smile disfigurement.

2. Good root planing can be uncomfortable for the patient. The deep areas of the periodontal pockets are infected with bacteria. Areas of infection are more acidic, and acid around the nerves in the gum tissue makes nerves more sensitive. The worse the infection, the more sensitive that area becomes, and the more uncomfortable the root planing is for a patient. Patients indicate to the hygienist that it hurts in that area and the hygienist may avoid properly measuring or cleaning to the depth of that infected site to keep their nice relationship with the patient (and perhaps keep their job by avoiding patient complaints to the dentist). Unfortunately, avoiding cleaning out the bacterial infection in the sensitive area eventually results in a tooth so diseased it must be extracted.

3. Most routine dental cleaning appointments are scheduled for the time to do a simple cleaning, but not for root planing or the unanticipated need for local anesthesia. Offices will often place a root planing appointment into a regular cleaning appointment length spot on the schedule. It takes time to administer local anesthesia and time for it to take effect. The unexpected need for local anesthesia to allow for treatment of sensitive periodontal pockets absorbs too much of the normal length cleaning appointment time to accomplish good root planing. This is irritating to everyone involved, except the bacteria!

4. Patients do not realize how important a separate root planing appointment is and are reluctant to want to receive an injection of local anesthesia to get the deep areas cleaned out.

5. Dentists often fail to refer patients to periodontists for root planing despite the fact that periodontal practices are usually the best at providing root planing. Periodontists are specialists in treating gum disease with root planing and surgery. Periodontists go for four years to dental school to become a dentist, then an additional three years to study just periodontics. A dentist loses income from their practice when referring a patient to a periodontist. In addition, dentists occasionally do not refer to periodontists for fear of losing the patient. This occurs sometimes when the patient hears how bad their gum disease is and realizes the referral for treatment should have occurred earlier.

6. If the dental hygienist cannot administer adequate local anesthesia, the dentist must be interrupted to give anesthesia (sometimes during a procedure by the dentist that cannot be stopped at that particular moment). This leads to procedures on two or more patients being delayed. This makes the dentist less happy with the hygienist. To avoid this situation, the hygienist may be less likely to address the most infected areas that need anesthesia to treat the disease well.

7. An additional reason why it is common for root planing to be done inadequately is dental practices can usually escape any ramifications for doing it quickly and poorly. They can get away with this reduction in quality treatment because it is difficult to determine whether root planing is done well at any particular appointment. If a patient does not stay at the same dental office for years, it is difficult to determine who is responsible for doing poor root planing that resulted in tooth loss.

8. Properly shaped instruments for each side of the tooth are necessary to do a complete removal of calculus and bacteria during root planing. This requires at least three differently shaped two-sided curettes on each root planing tray set up. Each curette costs $50.00 to $100.00. The curettes need to be sharp to do a good job. Nearly every time a curette is used it needs to be resharpened. Even running the curettes through the sterilizer dulls the instruments a little bit, resulting in a need to sharpen again. The sharpening means curettes wear out eventually and need to be replaced. Properly

replacing worn out curettes adds up to a significant additional part of an office's overhead expenses. This puts uncomfortable pressure on the hygienist to ask the dentist for new instruments. Avoiding asking for instrument replacements will result in poorer treatment.

9. A recent study showed over 60% of all dental offices do not properly probe and record the entire mouth on an annual basis as is required. This means the dentist and hygienist have no map of where to place their efforts or see what areas are getting worse. (It is not a coincidence that over half of all teeth are lost due to gum disease and over half of all dentists do not record full mouth periodontal probings each year.)

I know of a dentist who was doing a working interview at a corporate dental chain when he was asked to do root planing. The office had only one curette available, and one of the two sides of the curette was even broken off. No one could do good treatment with this instrument. It is important to go to an office where careful treatment is more important than corporate profits.

Takeaways

Unless the patient has already lost most of their teeth, it is highly improbable for a patient with moderate or advanced periodontal disease to get a proper full mouth of root planing in less than two to three hours. Most careful offices schedule at least forty-five minutes per one fourth (one quadrant) of the mouth.

If the office you frequent does a full mouth of root planing in an hour (often as part of a lump sum treatment quote), your health and pocketbook have been compromised.

Why don't antibiotics cure periodontitis?

Since bacteria are the main cause of gum disease and antibiotics help kill bacteria, why can't taking antibiotics cure gum disease?

When you take antibiotics, they get absorbed into your blood and float around in your major blood vessels and tiny capillaries. Capillary walls become porous and leaky when they are near tissue with bacterial infections. This allows your white blood cells to wiggle out of the capillaries and go fight the bacteria. Simultaneously, blood serum containing antibiotics also leak out with the white blood cells. The white blood cells and the antibiotics never reach the bacteria living in the center of large chunks of calculus. As soon as you quit taking the antibiotics, the remaining unaffected bacteria come out and continue to grow into big colonies and the progress of the periodontal disease resumes.

Scientific studies show that if the dentist or hygienist performs root planing to remove and disrupt the biofilm and calculus while the patient is simultaneously taking antibiotics, the periodontal therapy kills slightly more bacteria than just root planing. Unfortunately, the improvement in bacterial death with antibiotics is usually not very significant and should only be done if the periodontal disease has shown itself to be very difficult to eradicate.

Interestingly, this also explains why mouth rinses do not control periodontal disease. As long as your heart is pumping blood and you have infected periodontal pockets, the flow of serum coming out of the pockets and into your mouth creates a current strong enough to prevent mouth rinses and other fluids from flowing back down into the pockets. This is why mouthwash companies are prohibited from saying they treat periodontal disease, but they can say they address bacteria that is not under the gums and gingivitis which is an inflammation-only status not causing bone loss.

Antibiotics can pose risks

Another reason to avoid using antibiotics in treating gum disease is that the benefits they provide are low compared to the risks they pose to the patient, as described here:

1. Using antibiotics during root planing provides a marginal benefit at most and is extremely risky because of the possibility of allergic reactions.

2. Antibiotic usage has been proven to increase the number of bacteria that are resistant to the antibiotics. This reduces the benefit of antibiotics when needed for life-threatening issues.

3. More importantly, taking antibiotics increases the severe threat of disturbing the population of your normal protective intestinal organisms, leaving you susceptible to an infection from an increasingly common bacterium called *Clostridioides difficile*. This infection can be fatal. It causes bouts of severe bloody diarrhea and hospitalization. Clostridioides difficile infection has become a major cause of death in hospitals. Inserting fecal matter from healthy individuals into a sick person's intestines to provide new healthy bacteria has become a common treatment for this terrible disease.

Periodontal disease may magnify other disease processes

Numerous systemic issues are correlated with periodontal disease. We believe this is because the body's response to gum disease bacteria causes the capillary walls to be porous and leaky. When you chew with teeth that have gum disease, bacteria can be pumped into adjacent leaky capillaries and into the bloodstream. Coughing can also cause aerosolized bacteria laden saliva droplets to get into in the lungs. Numerous scientific journal articles show the following disease states have been linked to gum disease:

- atherosclerosis
- thrombosis
- myocardial infarction
- stroke (gum disease bacteria are often found in the site of brain abscesses)
- pneumonia
- chronic obstructive pulmonary disease
- rheumatoid arthritis
- mothers having preterm birth and low birth weight babies

- diabetes
- kidney, lung, pancreas, oral, throat, and blood cancers
- poorer nutrition
- possible poorer overall cancer surveillance due to an overworked immune system
- poorer response to Covid and other diseases

Spreading excessive amounts of periodontal pathogenic bacteria throughout the body is a serious threat in many ways. It can cause an increase in generalized inflammation that is associated with many diseases. Besides oral bacteria being found in the blockage area of stroke victims, over 30 different types of cancer have been shown to harbor bacteria associated with and living in the cancerous tumors. *Fusobacterium nucleatum*, a periodontal disease bacterium that has been found in breast cancer samples, may damage our ability to fight the cancer. These bacteria make a protein that binds to our immune cells and can block those cells from destroying cancer cells. The fact that gum disease is associated with all these diseases makes diagnosing and treating it even more important.

Periodontal surgery

Periodontal surgery may need to be performed if scaling and root planing fails to resolve the periodontal infection. Remaining infection is determined by redness, bleeding, and sometimes pus. If you still have bleeding pockets 5 mm or greater after root planing, it means bacteria are still present in grooves or root irregularities. If this is the case, you may need to have periodontal surgery to remove those bacteria and control the infection. This is especially true if you have already lost a few teeth to periodontal disease.

Periodontal surgery is done to eliminate the causes of periodontal disease and reduce the depth of the pockets. Healthier tissue will make it easier to remove bacteria at home and at subsequent professional visits. Removing the damaging bacteria will reduce future bone and tooth loss, especially if followed by good oral hygiene and dental cleanings every three months.

During periodontal surgery, the gums are incised with a scalpel and are pushed back to see the roots. The roots are cleaned and special efforts are made to reach the hard-to-access areas where the roots start to divide and have grooves. Periodontal surgery can also be done to reduce pocket depths by reshaping the jawbone and regenerating bone and tissue.

Periodontal surgery has been proven to help you keep your teeth significantly longer than letting periodontal disease fester. The greatest benefit is obtained after periodontal surgery if you have good oral hygiene and strict adherence to periodontal maintenance cleanings every three months. Three months is a magic number for most people. It takes about three months after a good cleaning for the bacteria to sneak back under the gums and re-establish themselves in a virulent and large enough group to start the bone loss again.

Many patients ask about laser-based periodontal therapy as an alternative treatment since it does not have as many side effects as traditional scalpel-based surgery. Laser-based periodontal therapy does not eliminate the deep spaces that allow anaerobic bacteria regrow as well as traditional surgery. Lasers are an excellent tool for some uses, such as root canal treatment, tissue shape changes, and treating failing implants, but it appears to me that laser-based periodontitis treatment is not as effective as traditional scalpel-based periodontal surgery. More than twenty-five years of research has proven that laser-based periodontal therapy is about as valuable as scaling and root planing and is no substitute for traditional periodontal surgery. (Cobb CM Lasers and the treatment of periodontitis; the essence and the noise. Periodontol 2000. 2017; 75:205-295). Make sure to see who paid for the research and evaluate what their motivation is when you read any article or advertisement regarding the benefits of laser surgery or other therapy. When evaluating laser therapy for periodontitis, of nearly 500 possibly eligible articles, fewer than 30 met the criterion for review for a proper meta-analysis. This combined analysis showed a periodontal pocket depth benefit of root planing plus laser surgery versus root planing alone of less than one millimeter. Overall, this is an extremely modest improvement at best, but occasionally individual tooth results can be much better. This means to me more frequent root planing by an excellent dental hygienist may be the clear cost-effective way to help control gum disease. Search for up-to-date truths about laser surgery at the American Academy of Periodontology website or aap.onlinelibrary.wiley.com.

In my opinion, studies supporting laser-based periodontal therapy need to be several years longer than currently available to evaluate if laser surgery prevents the reestablishment of progressive periodontal disease. Of course, scientific analysis can change therapies over time.

My book is informational and designed to be a consumer advocacy resource, so the undesirable aspects of every therapy are presented to allow the reader to fully understand each therapy. There are decades of clear evidence that scalpel-based traditional periodontal surgery helps keep your teeth, but there are some negative side effects to this historically proven periodontal surgery which are discussed below.

Negative side effects of periodontal surgery

Bleeding. It is common for some bleeding to occur after periodontal surgery is performed. The local anesthesia injected to numb the tissues during periodontal surgery contains blood vessel constricting components (usually epinephrine). The blood vessels in the surgical area are constricted and therefore less blood flows through the area. Because there is less blood flowing through the area, the anesthetic liquid deposited is not washed away and the anesthesia lasts longer. Blood vessel constricting components make the anesthesia last much longer without needing new injections.

Your body knows the blood vessels have been constricted and tries to make up for the reduced blood flow by dilating the vessels larger than normal after the anesthesia wears off. This increased blood vessel diameter sends more blood and oxygen to the area once again when the vessel constricting component wears off.

This temporary extra blood flow is great for wound healing, but after surgery you can experience a disconcerting sudden gush of blood from the surgical site for a few minutes to an hour before the blood vessels shrink back to normal.

Once the initial anesthesia wears off and the blood vessels get back to normal, there can be some normal minor oozing of blood that can last from one to three days.

Temperature sensitivity. Temperature sensitivity is a common negative result associated with most periodontal surgeries. This is because periodontal surgery often exposes some of the root structure.

The crown of the tooth is the part of the tooth you see when you smile, and it is covered with enamel. Enamel does not contain nerves, so it is not sensitive to temperature. The roots of the teeth are made of dentin and have nerve endings down the middle of the tooth and throughout the tooth extending to the edges of the root. The new position of the gums after periodontal surgery exposes some of the root and nerve endings so you may feel cold fluids, hot fluids, and even cold air.

I have an example of this sensitivity with a patient who always rode a motorcycle to my office. He rode it even on a particularly cold day when I removed his sutures and protective dressings covering his gums and teeth a week after surgery. After the appointment, he left the office on his motorcycle and promptly turned around to come back to the office. He waited in my office for his wife to bring his motorcycle helmet with a face shield to protect his teeth from the discomfort caused by cold air. Fortunately, the cold sensitivity resolved in a few weeks due to his great oral hygiene and a prescription fluoride toothpaste.

This type of bothersome temperature sensitivity will diminish rapidly if the teeth roots are kept clean of bacteria with great toothbrushing efforts. Sensitivity can also be controlled with over-the-counter toothpastes formulated for sensitive teeth or by prescription fluoride. A special effort with tooth brushing must be made to clean the teeth thoroughly. Then fluoride, the ingredients in desensitizing toothpastes, or even salts in the saliva will plug up the tiny tubules in the root to block the nerve endings from feeling temperature changes.

New cavities can occur on roots. Tooth roots are composed of dentin, which is not as hard as the enamel of natural crowns. The softness of root dentin means the acid produced by bacteria can dissolve the root quicker than the crown. Therefore, roots are much more likely to get cavities. Periodontal surgery repositions the gumline to reduce the depth of the spaces (pockets) where bacteria hide from our brushing efforts. Root surfaces can be exposed when the gumline is changed.

Care must be taken to prevent dental cavities from forming on the roots. Most of us have a regular tendency of brushing our teeth in a straight line where the teeth have always been. If you keep brushing in a straight line after the gum height has been changed and root exposed, it is easy to miss areas where the roots are newly exposed after surgery. To prevent cavities, special efforts must be made to brush bacteria off these newly exposed root surfaces. Electric oscillating round-headed toothbrushes like those from Oral-B® can help hit all these areas. Additionally, both interproximal brushes that slide between the teeth and water flossers are excellent to remove bacteria growing on surfaces between the roots. Fluoride and molecular iodine mouth rinses, prescription fluoride applications, and fluoride toothpastes can also help prevent cavities from forming.

Negative esthetic impact. The gums shrink after periodontal surgery and the teeth often look longer. This usually results in a negative esthetic impact. Almost everyone agrees, however, it is better to have longer teeth than teeth no longer!

Empty spaces are created between the teeth. The entire root of a tooth is generally shaped like a snow cone (triangular with the tip of the triangle being the tip of the root). Therefore, when the gums are repositioned further towards the root tips, spaces are created between the teeth. This is particularly irritating because the extra triangular spaces between the teeth can hold pieces of food.

In addition, cosmetic research tells us that the most negative appearance flaw in a smile is any dark shadow. Every triangular space created by the gum missing between roots creates a dark shadow area.

The visible small empty spaces between teeth are irritating, but losing entire teeth is a bigger esthetic concern. Eliminating these triangular spaces with crowns, white fillings or gum augmentation is occasionally performed.

Discomfort. There is pain and soreness for five to ten days after periodontal surgery. To best control this discomfort make sure you start taking the analgesic (ibuprofen or other drug) *before* the numbness (anesthetic) wears off. If you like to minimize taking any drugs, do not try to convince yourself that you are tough and are going to be fine with the pain. In the end, you will be taking more drugs if you do not address the potential pain before the anesthesia wears off.

Scientific studies show there are physiologic changes in the nerve channels that allow more perfect conduction of pain once pain occurs. This means if you allow yourself to get very sore before trying to get rid of pain, the changes in the nerves will make the pain more intense and linger longer before the situation improves. It takes days for the sensitized nerve channels to get back to normal. The message here is to take your pain medications before the numbness wears off.

Infection. There is a small risk (less than 10%) of infection after periodontal surgery. If you have medical issues that make you more prone to infection, it could be higher for you.

Throughout our six million years of evolution, we were exposed to bone, dirt, sand, sharp twigs, and other abrasive objects inside of our food. This meant we would often scratch and cut up our mouths when eating certain meals. The individuals with strong localized immune system responses fought off these bacterial and virus-laden injuries better than those who did not have immediate and strong immune protection.

Evolving and improving over time, humans eventually developed a dense tonsillar ring of immune cell producing lymphoid tissue around the inside of our throat (Waldeyer's ring). These lymphoid tissues include palatal, throat, and tongue tonsils surrounding the mouth and throat. They produce the white blood cells that fight infection, providing us an immediate and voluminous army of white blood cells to attack any foreign bodies that penetrate the skin of the mouth. This beneficial dense ring of immune protection helps rapid healing in the mouth and minimizes infection after periodontal surgery.

Periodontal disease can reoccur despite surgery. Studies show you will get recurrent periodontal disease if you do not see the dental hygienist every two to four months and develop excellent daily brushing and flossing habits. The research clearly shows periodontal disease gets worse faster if you visit the dental hygienist only every six months rather than visiting the dental hygienist every three months. Unfortunately, most standard dental insurance plans only pay for dental cleanings twice yearly. Dental insurance companies are aware of the need for patients with periodontal disease to have dental cleanings four times a year and some offer premium plans with this provision.

At first blush, it seems to matter very little if you stretch your regularly scheduled dental cleaning appointments out from three months to four months. Thinking about the following scenario, however, underscores the importance of seeing a hygienist every three months instead of every four months. The following situation is actually fairly accurate for most people with periodontal disease.

Imagine that after a good dental cleaning, you have no damage occurring in your gums until the bacteria in your periodontal pockets evolve into a big enough colony of the aggressive, oxygen-hating bacteria. This happens for most people at around ninety days (three months). If you wait for a cleaning until four months has passed, the infection has been destroying your bone for thirty days. This destruction can add up. If you follow the same four-month cleaning schedule for a year, you have lost bone for three total months as compared to almost none at all if you saw a good hygienist every three months. Clinically, we also see most patients have gums that bleed much more at a four-month cleaning interval than if the same patient comes in after three months. This situation is even more obvious at six-month intervals.

Bruising and swelling. Bruising and swelling are common after periodontal surgery. Bruising is usually resolved in a week to ten days. Swelling is usually the worst at three to four days, then rapidly resolves.

Soft tissue graft issues. Sometimes soft tissue graft periodontal surgery is done to cover up exposed roots and place tougher gum tissue to reduce future recession. These procedures are occasionally not esthetically perfect due to bulkiness and/or occasional incomplete root coverage, but they are a reliable improvement. Also, roots covered by healthy gums are much less likely to get cavities.

> **Takeaways**
>
> Your biggest risk of tooth loss is usually periodontal disease. You must have a good periodontal exam to know your gum health status. If you are not getting annual periodontal probing exams at your dental cleanings, that is a big red flag. Asking for a copy of your periodontal probing exam is a nonconfrontational way to help keep your teeth by helping to ensure your dental hygienist and dentist are paying attention to gum disease. Requesting a written document of your periodontal health forces them to try to be accurate when creating your periodontal charting and pay closer attention to teeth in trouble.

Deep periodontal pockets and associated loss of bone supporting the teeth result in loose, ugly teeth surrounded by red, bleeding gums and eventual tooth loss.

Ideally, active periodontal therapy like root planing with local anesthesia should begin at 5 mm to avoid this ticking time bomb of disease progression from getting to dangerous depths. Unfortunately, you get no warning that tooth loss is imminent because even at 8 mm gum disease is not usually painful. Warning: Do not fail to get treatment if your pocket is 8 mm or deeper even if your dentist suggests to just "watch" the area. This is when you really need excellent root planing and seeing a periodontist may provide you with your best chance at saving the teeth.

Despite some of the discomfort associated with periodontal surgery, keeping your natural teeth for the long haul is an overwhelmingly positive reason to consider surgery. Plus, over a lifetime, keeping your natural teeth is usually far less expensive than tooth replacement procedures like implants and bridges. (Bernadette Pretzl et al. J Clin Periodontol. 2009 Aug.)

Two

Dental Fillings

Dental fillings are used to replace damaged tooth structure. Tooth structure may need to be replaced because of cavities (dental caries) or other damage to the tooth. The materials used for dental fillings are tooth-colored composites or silver and mercury amalgam. There are benefits and disadvantages of each filling material.

Tooth-Colored Dental Fillings

Dentists use the terms "tooth-colored dental fillings" and "composites" interchangeably. These are resins that harden in response to light and chemical reactions. They contain methacrylate monomers and fillers that are either quartz or glass. The fillers are included to resist abrasion from chewing pressures because the resin material by itself is somewhat soft and wears down easily.

The positives and negatives

Tooth-colored dental fillings are made to match the color of a natural tooth. These composite fillings can restore damaged tooth structure or be added to improve the shape of a deficient tooth. They are an excellent choice for many tooth restorations.

Composite restorations can look great, but there are some negative aspects of these tooth-colored fillings, as noted below:

Failures. Composite restorations can fail sometimes due to cavities forming around the filling. Results are technique sensitive: to avoid a poor result the dentist must follow a precise series of steps. There are many more steps for placing a composite restoration than there are for placing an amalgam filling. Furthermore, the process requires a precise number of seconds for each step and the tooth needs to remain dry for materials to bond and harden properly. For example, the tooth is etched with an acid and if this acid is on the tooth too long or too briefly, then the filling will not adhere as strongly.

Inadequate hardening. Most composite fillings need to be hardened with a special light. This light will not harden several millimeters deep of composite at once. The light is turned on in steps as the space in the tooth is filled up a few millimeters at a time. This ensures each layer has hardened adequately. Failure to follow the composite manufacturer's instructions may result in inadequate hardening and can cause the filling to fail or fall out. It is also important to pay attention to details because each brand of composite can have different time requirements. Some studies have even shown that cheap dental lights do not harden the composite filling as deeply as promised by the manufacturer. Going to a low-cost, high volume dental office can place you at risk for these problems.

Less compression strength. Large composite fillings on back teeth cannot resist strong chewing forces as well as silver amalgam fillings. Grinding on these teeth may cause cracks. A composite filling may also crack because the filling did not have enough depth in certain areas.

Clinical problem of shrinkage. One of the main clinical problems with composite fillings revolves around the shrinkage of the composite as it hardens at the initial placement appointment. This shrinkage can result in several problems:

1. Shrinkage pressures can cause tiny gaps as areas of the composite break away from the tooth enamel at the connection of the composite and the tooth. This tiny gap can create microleakage resulting in sensitivity, new cavity formation, and staining in the gap.

2. The shrinkage can also leave a tiny gap deep inside the hole that the filling filled, which can cause sensitivity.

Chemical ingredient concerns. Bisphenol A (BPA) derivatives (bis-GMA, bis-DMA, bis-EMA, bis-MPEPP, PC bis-GMA) are found in dental composites. Holistic and biologic dentists point out these BPA compounds are toxic. But these compounds enhance the longevity of composites. It has not been demonstrated if the small dosage of exposure to these products can cause disease.

Despite these problems, tooth-colored filling materials remain an excellent choice for tooth restorations.

Composite fillings for root notches

Roots are softer than the tooth enamel. If roots are exposed, brushing teeth with hard toothbrush bristles or abrasive toothpastes can create notches in the roots. Dental fillings (usually the tooth-colored type) are done in these notches to stop abrasion before the nerve in the center of the tooth is exposed. In addition, it is prudent to do the protective filling before the tooth becomes so worn away that the tooth may risk being snapped in half when biting on hard food. Notches in the roots can also be caused by hard biting forces exceeding root strength.

Unfortunately, if these side-of-tooth fillings are not done soon enough, notching in the roots can lead to sensitivity and eventually a need for a root canal if the wear gets too close to the nerve.

Amalgam Silver Fillings

Silver-colored dental fillings are called amalgam. Amalgam is 50% mercury by weight. Most of the rest of amalgam is silver, tin, and copper. There are also small amounts of zinc, palladium, and indium.

The positive features

Amalgam is a *long-lasting restoration* material, and *amalgam fillings can be placed in an area that cannot be kept dry.* Water disrupts the hardening and adhesion of tooth-colored composites.

Unfortunately, there are some negative aspects of using amalgam for fillings.

The negatives

Unesthetic. Amalgam is a shiny silver color and that makes it among the least esthetic of the dental restoration materials. Many dental practices do not use amalgam anymore because it does not look appealing.

Metal conducts heat and electricity. Amalgam is a metal, so it can conduct temperature changes to the nerve in the center of the tooth. This sometimes results in hot and cold sensitivity.

Allergy. Some individuals can have an allergy or sensitivity to any of the components of dental amalgam. This is a good reason not to get amalgam fillings, although this situation is rare.

Mercury. Exposure to high levels of mercury vapor is associated with adverse health effects in the brain and the kidneys. However, the United States Food and Drug Administration has determined that dental amalgam fillings containing mercury are safe for adults and children ages six and above. There is no peer-reviewed scientific evidence that shows the amount of mercury in dental fillings causes medical issues in the general population.

Many individuals wish to avoid mercury-containing amalgam dental fillings to minimize any risk that is discovered in the future. It is well known that mercury from any source (commonly fish) can build up over time in your body's organs or tissues, especially in the brain and kidneys. But this type of mercury that builds up in fish (methylmercury) is not the same type of mercury found in dental amalgam.

Despite the science that demonstrates that amalgam fillings are safe, it may be recommended that some individuals avoid the mercury in amalgam fillings. That would include pregnant women or women planning on getting pregnant, nursing mothers, unborn babies, children under six, people with a mercury allergy, kidney dysfunction, or neurological impairment (for a complete list see FDA.gov).

Removing amalgam fillings

Some people want to remove their amalgam fillings. It has been proved that the amount of mercury released or ingested when removing an amalgam filling is higher than the amount that is released over the entire lifetime of a patient who chooses to keep amalgam fillings in place.

> **Takeaways**
>
> More tooth structure is removed each time a filling is replaced. The fewer times you replace a dental filling over the course of your life, the greater the likelihood of keeping your teeth.
>
> Tooth-colored fillings are usually the recommended option because of their advantages. However, tooth-colored composites are technique-sensitive and do not do well when the dentist cannot keep the tooth dry enough during the placement of the filling. There are also white "glass ionomer" and similar materials that are used in situations when it is difficult to keep the tooth dry during placement.

Three

Crowns

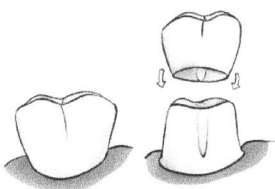

Figure 3.1 Original undisturbed tooth (left) and prepared tooth and crown (right).

A crown is a cap that covers all or most of the visible portion of your tooth. Crowns are often necessary to replace teeth partially destroyed by cavities and fractures. Crowns are also done to improve esthetics and supply structural support to a tooth that invariably becomes brittle after root canals.

Some of your tooth structure needs to be removed to create room for a crown to slide over the top of your remaining natural tooth. The tooth needs to be shaped like a tapered water cup so a crown can slide over the tooth and be cemented on. (See Figure3.1.) A dentist must grind away tooth material to taper the tooth.

Crowns on natural teeth have a good long-term prognosis. Around 85% of crowns will last fifteen years. When they do fail, it is usually because of dental cavities.

Know the Pros and Cons

Despite dental crowns having a very promising prognosis, there are some risks and concerns that you should understand before having a crown procedure.

Your dentist should make sure the tooth nerve is healthy before a crown is placed. Your dentist should take an x-ray that shows the tip of the root (periapical x-ray) to check the health of the tooth. Other ways to test for tooth health include ice or electrical tests. These tests can help the dentist determine if a root canal is needed *before* the crown is done.

If a tooth is not healthy and needs a root canal, then the root canal should be done before doing a crown. After a crown is placed, sometimes it is determined that the nerve is not healthy. If this happens, the root canal procedure is performed by drilling a hole in the crown. A crown should last fifteen or more years, but a crown with a hole in it is likely to fail much sooner. Here are some reasons why:

To perform a root canal, a hole is drilled in the top of the natural tooth or crown. This hole will irreparably damage a crown. The crown will be patched with filling material, but the surface irregularity between the crown and filling can occasionally lead to bacteria and food getting in over time. This is especially true when compared to the pristine smooth surface of a new crown. And another problem with the border between these two different materials is they expand and contract to temperature changes by a different amount. This "thermal expansion" causes small gaps at the border, allowing bacteria to grow into the gaps and create a cavity. Also, a cavity in that location is impossible to see in an x-ray and can increase in size undetected and lead to tooth loss.

It is sad to say, but it is common to see a crown placed on a tooth that should have had a root canal first. I have personally seen more than a thousand examples where x-ray evidence prior to the crown shows the patient should have had a root canal done before a crown was placed, but a root canal was not done. What often happens is the dentist addresses what they believe is the main issue, which is the tooth that is broken or has a cavity. But in focusing on the physical loss of tooth structure, they may overlook the health of the nerve.

Even under the best of circumstances, the trauma of trimming down the tooth in preparation for a crown can kill the tooth. Numerous scientific papers report at least 15% of crown preparations create this issue and result in needing a root canal. Nevertheless, checking the health of the tooth before getting the crown done can minimize this risk of needing to pay for a second crown on the same tooth shortly after a root canal.

Occasionally, patients are their own worst enemy because they do not know about these issues and refuse an extra x-ray to check for tooth health before a crown is made. One extra x-ray taken before a crown can prevent needing a second crown, eventually more additional x-rays, and possible tooth loss in the future. Keeping your teeth is too important to go to any dentist who works as fast as possible to produce maximum profit every day. *Ask the dentist to check the nerve health before rushing to do a crown.*

Choosing the crown material

Crowns can be made of several different kinds of materials. The choice of crown material can affect appearance, microscopic fit, speed of production, risk of allergic reaction, and amount of healthy tooth that needs to be removed. In addition, the choice of crown material also affects the chance of wear or chipping on opposing teeth.

Tooth-colored crowns are made from white solid material or white material attached to a metal substructure. Tooth-colored crowns require the removal of more tooth structure than gold or metal crowns. Tooth-colored crown material needs to be thicker to be strong and to look natural. You also get closer to the center of the tooth because more tooth structure is removed to make room for the thicker crown. Since more tooth structure must be removed, more friction and heat are created. The nerve and blood vessels in the center of the tooth are very heat-sensitive. Any extra tooth structure removal increases thermal damage risk and increases root canal likelihood.

It is worth knowing just how hard these tooth-colored crowns are. Zirconia is the most common tooth-colored crown material and just half a millimeter of zirconia is ten times harder than concrete. So, crowns will always chip or wear opposing teeth more than a filling will and this is especially relevant for front teeth. Getting an unnecessary front crown instead of a filling can lead to chipping the opposing tooth over time or suddenly, when you trip, for example, and your teeth come together sharply.

If esthetics is not a concern (such as with a back tooth), choosing a gold or noble metal crown can help you preserve your teeth by minimizing thermal damage, retaining more tooth structure, and minimizing the risk of needing a root canal.

Crown color is permanent. The color of the crown or filling made by your dentist is permanent and cannot be whitened after placement. If you end up wanting to get your teeth whitened, your natural teeth will get lighter in color, but the crowns made by your dentist will not change color. This also applies to tooth-colored fillings, bridges, and other dental work. If you are planning on whitening your teeth, the general recommendation is that you should do the whitening before crowns or new fillings. That way your color chosen for new crowns and fillings will be made with a whiter material to match your newly whitened natural teeth. The exception, however, is if you have open cavities. The bleaching liquid can go into the cavity and give you significant sharp pain while bleaching and may damage the tooth. Your dentist can advise you on the sequence for your individual situation.

Crown shape

A new crown should usually match the size and shape of the original tooth (unless the original tooth is malformed or badly positioned). Sometimes the crown is made so that it is a little bulkier than the original natural tooth shape. This over-contoured area where the tooth touches the crown can trap bacteria leading to cavities and periodontal disease. On the other hand, if the crown is made under-contoured, or it does not fit closely to the prepared edge of the natural tooth, food and bacteria accumulate at this junction and can cause cavities and periodontal disease.

Risk during procedure

The grinding on a tooth with a dental bur during the procedure creates friction that heats up the tooth. The nerve and pulp tissue in the center of the tooth can be injured or die if there is too much heat created. This injury can be painful and may necessitate a root canal. If the nerve dies, then eventually the dead nerve tissue leaks out through the root tip into the jawbone. You can see evidence of dead nerves by looking at an x-ray. Bone disappears because white blood cells from your bloodstream attack and dissolve dead tissue, bacteria, and part of your jawbone in the area. The jawbone is an innocent bystander. Missing bone appears on an x-ray as a dark spot at the tip or side of the tooth's root. This dark spot indicates you need a root canal to remove the dead material and bacteria from the center of the tooth.

The dentist sprays cool water on the tooth during the crown procedure to minimize the amount of heat created when trimming down the tooth. Despite efforts by the dentist to keep the tooth cool, thermal damage leads to a minimum of 15% of all crowned teeth eventually having the pulps die and needing root canals. An additional risk is drying out and damaging the live tooth by leaving the trimmed down tooth exposed to room air and/or spraying on the tooth for too many minutes. It takes a skilled dentist to balance taking enough time to properly trim down the tooth to make an ideal shape for a crown, but not so long as to excessively traumatize the tooth.

Veneers versus Crowns

Veneers are surface replacements or coverings on mainly the visible side of a tooth to improve the appearance, color, or shape of less-than-ideal teeth. Veneers are made with filling material or tooth-colored ceramic material like the materials used in crowns. But veneers are thinner and less sturdy than crowns. This is good because the dentist can take off less tooth structure than a crown requires, however, minimal tooth removal can leave a tiny edge of the veneer that sticks out beyond the tooth surface. This raised edge can retain bacteria. These bacteria can cause the gums around the veneer to get red and inflamed. Another negative aspect of the thinness of the veneer means it is more likely to chip or break down at the margins and need to be replaced. In other words, crowns go all the way around a tooth and therefore are sturdier than veneers. Veneers are very technique-sensitive because they rely less on 360 degrees of cement helping them stay on and more on every step of preparation and bonding being done correctly. Because veneers are often the most fragile of all dental restorations, you are likely to be replacing them more often.

Takeaway

Despite the risks and issues described above, dental crowns generally have long lives and are mandatory in many situations. Single-tooth crowns placed on natural teeth often last more than fifteen years. Crowns that are placed on dental implants also have excellent prognoses with most single-tooth implant crowns lasting more than ten years if the implant has not failed first.

Four

Bridges/Fixed Partial Dentures

What Is a Bridge?

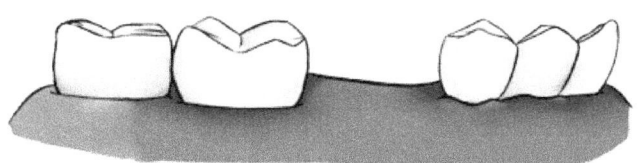

Figure 4.1. Missing lower tooth.

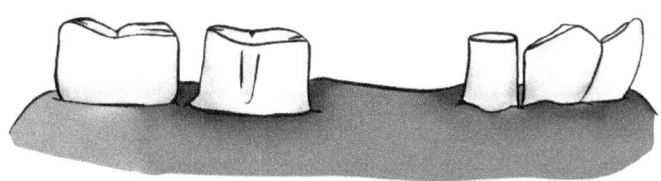

Figure 4.2. Teeth prepared (trimmed down for bridge).

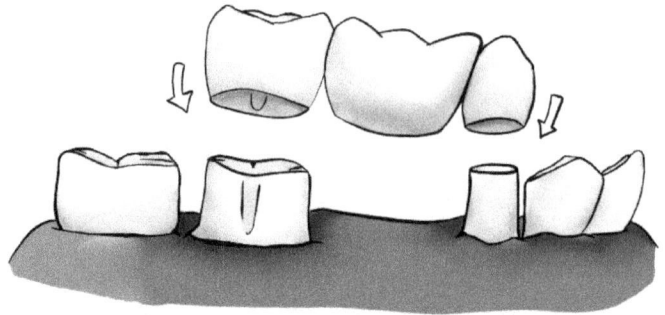

Figure 4.3. A bridge slides onto and is cemented over prepared teeth.

A bridge is made to replace one or more missing teeth. It is a single piece with one or more crowns on each end and a fake tooth or teeth in the middle. (See Figure 4.3.) A bridge slides over what remains of the natural teeth on each end. This bridge is glued or "cemented" onto teeth that have been trimmed down. The term "fixed partial denture" is another name for bridges that are permanently attached by glue, cement, or screws to implants or to natural teeth. The patient cannot remove them. (Bridges and fixed partial dentures are the same, and I will use the term "bridges" in this chapter.)

Bridges are often an excellent choice to replace missing teeth, especially if bone in the area is not adequate in size or quality to hold an implant. Replacing teeth with a bridge is often faster than using implants. Bridges are a predictable treatment, and nearly 75% of all bridges last ten years. However, bridges can occasionally fail.

Why Bridges Fail

Bridges can fail sooner than individual crowns, but some of these failures can be minimized or delayed by understanding the reasons for their failure and instituting proper home care and timely dental visits.

Cavities

Dental cavities are the most common reason for bridges to fail. Bridges have a fake tooth that blocks easy access for toothbrush bristles or floss from easily cleaning bacteria and food away from the natural and fake tooth surfaces. This makes decay form quicker. It is important to keep up with your scheduled dental visits if you have a bridge so the area can be cleaned well and early problems can be resolved simply.

Tooth preparation trauma

The teeth supporting bridges can be lost for the same reasons that teeth are lost after crowns are placed on them (fractures, cavities, etc.), but bridges also pose additional risk to the teeth.

Because there are at least two teeth involved, the failure rate for bridges is more than twice as high as it is for a simple crown. Bridges are one solid piece and need at least one tooth supporting either end of the bridge to be trimmed down in preparation for crown placement. As was discussed earlier, each new crown has a 15% risk of its vital supporting tooth needing a root canal from the thermal damage caused by trimming down the tooth to make room for the crown to slide on top of the tooth. A bridge is glued onto at least two teeth, so it needs the creation of a minimum of two crown preparations. Because a bridge involves at least two teeth, the risk of needing a root canal access hole drilled into and damaging a brand-new bridge increases to a 30% chance.

Teeth drift or tilt if missing teeth are not replaced

If a missing tooth is not replaced quickly, teeth adjacent to where a tooth is missing can drift or tilt into that missing tooth's space. This causes two problems:

1. A tilted tooth does not handle biting forces well—it's like a roof supported by a tilted wall. Teeth handle biting forces best when teeth are in a normal vertical position. This is especially important when a bridge replaces missing teeth since the associated extra pressure from the span of the unsupported missing tooth is placed on the tilted teeth.

2. The crowns on both ends of the bridge still need to slide straight down even if placed on a tilted tooth. A tilted tooth needs to be trimmed down to a greater degree on one side than the other side. This causes the trimming of the tooth to get closer to the nerve, blood vessel, and pulp on one side. (See Figure 4.4.) Trimming the tooth closer to the sensitive nerve in the center creates heat and mechanical trauma and increases the risk of killing the nerve and needing a root canal on the tilted tooth.

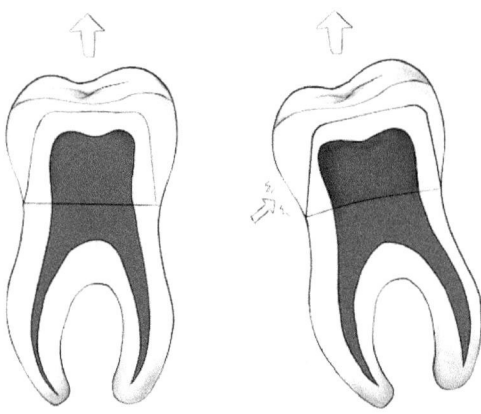

Figure 4.4. Trimming a tilted tooth so a crown will slide on gets close to the nerve.

Sometimes orthodontic braces are needed to tip the tilted tooth back into its vertical position before doing a crown for a bridge. This should eliminate the two problems listed above and increase the likelihood of keeping the tooth healthy. This type of orthodontics to upright a single tooth can be much quicker and less expensive than full braces.

Difficulties in cleaning

With a bridge in place, there is no way to floss around the fake tooth or teeth except by sliding floss underneath the bridge. This adds to the time needed to completely clean the teeth. In addition to a toothbrush, you might use an interproximal brush, special yarn, or bridge threaders to make it easier to clean underneath the bridge. Being unable to clean under the bridge results in cavities, the need for a new bridge, and possibly losing the supporting teeth.

Extra pressure on remaining teeth

Even when the bridge is perfectly made, we are asking the two natural teeth supporting the bridge to handle the chewing and biting forces that originally were distributed over three or four teeth. This increases the risk of the natural teeth being exposed to too much force and can lead to fracture or increased risk of periodontal disease. Dental implants are an option to avoid the overloading of natural teeth that can occur with bridges. An implant is also a good choice because it stands alone and you do not damage the adjacent teeth through trauma and risks of tooth preparation and extra biting pressures on perfectly healthy teeth that will occur with a bridge.

Takeaways

If you lose a tooth, make sure to promptly fill the space to avoid additional problems in the future. If the teeth on either side of the empty space are in perfect shape and do not need any dentistry done, a dental implant may be the best choice.

Five

Removable Partial Dentures

A removable partial denture is a single prosthetic piece with premade teeth that rests on your gums and remaining teeth. It is designed to replace several missing teeth with one device. A removable partial denture slides in and out between the remaining teeth and can clasp onto them. You take it out to clean it daily and leave it out at night. Bridges (also called fixed partial dentures) differ from removable partial dentures because bridges are permanently attached to the teeth.

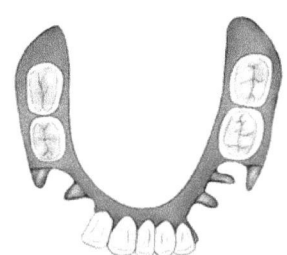

Figure 5.1. A removable partial denture.

A removable partial denture helps keep your remaining teeth from shifting, helps support your lips, helps you chew, and can improve your appearance. Removable partial denture fabrication for several teeth at once can be a quicker and less expensive choice than crowns, bridges, or implants. If you need several crowns and cannot afford them, you can have those defective teeth extracted and have a removable partial denture made and replace all the teeth at once.

Reasons for Choosing Removable Partial Dentures

Removable partial dentures offer certain practical advantages for some patients to replace missing teeth. Here are some:

Financial. Removable partial dentures are much less costly than most other treatment choices. And removable partial dentures usually do not get much more expensive when more missing teeth are being replaced, so they are a good choice when many spaces are being filled this way.

Lack of room for implants. Removable partial dentures may be a better choice when you do not have enough height or width of bone to do implants.

Temporary functional and esthetic replacement of teeth. Removable partial dentures can provide temporary functional and esthetic replacement of teeth while waiting for the body to heal after implant placement, extractions, cancer surgery, traumatic injury, or a bone regeneration procedure.

To save time and number of appointments. A removable partial denture can replace many missing teeth scattered around the same arch at one time. Removable partial dentures can save time and reduce the number of appointments.

Immediate time constraints. When you need to have many teeth replaced rapidly for an upcoming wedding, job interview, family gathering, or important event where you need to look your best, removable partial denture fabrication can be quicker than other options.

Avoiding discomfort. There is almost no postoperative discomfort associated with fabrication and placement of removable partial dentures, when there could be postoperative discomfort with crowns, bridges, or implants.

Advantages over fixed partial bridges. For some patients *removable* partial bridges offer additional advantages over *fixed* partial bridges, including the following:

1. Your good teeth may be too far apart to place a permanently cemented bridge because it will flex too much and fail if the space between the teeth is too great.

2. A removable partial denture can be the best choice when you are missing the teeth on the corner of your arch, such as your canines. Your jaw is naturally curved at the corners. If you lose a corner tooth, a bridge must curve out over where the corner tooth is missing in order to support the lips. If the bridge does not curve out and support your lips, your cheek will fall into that area and cause wrinkles. If you make a bridge with fake teeth curving outwards to support your lips, this central part of the curve has no tooth directly under the outward most point of the curve. This creates an unsupported cantilever. If you bite down on the outer curve of the bridge that is not supported by a tooth, the forces can break your teeth that are holding the bridge or break the cement loose that is holding the bridge to the teeth.

3. A removable partial denture has a large surface that covers and rests on the gums where teeth are missing to distribute biting forces more evenly. Using the gum ridge for support, a removable partial denture can handle the stress of the forces of chewing better than a permanently cemented bridge out over the edge of a curve.

4. A removable partial denture may be a better choice when the teeth on either side of the area of missing teeth are too weak or too short to support a permanently cemented bridge.

5. If you are missing teeth all the way in the back of your mouth, there is nothing on which to attach the back portion of a permanently cemented bridge. Whereas a removable partial denture can be supported solely by your gums in the back of your mouth.

Negative Aspects of Removable Partial Dentures

As with all medical and dental therapies, there are negative aspects that should be measured against the positive aspects. This is particularly advisable when you are considering removable partial dentures. Here are the main negative aspects of this therapy:

Survival rate. Removable partial dentures are initially inexpensive. Unfortunately, they have an approximate 40% survival rate at five years and

20% survival rate at ten years. Their reduced survival rate is partly because removable partial dentures exert pressure upon and slowly loosen the supporting natural teeth. Increased rates of decay and gum disease are also seen on the supporting teeth.

Bone loss. Your jaw loses bone more quickly under the partial denture because biting causes constant pressure on the gums. If you lose too much bone, then you lose support for your removable partial dentures.

Less bone can limit implant options. Enough vertical bone height above vital structures such as nerves is required to place implants. If you lose bone under a removable partial denture, you may not have enough bone to do dental implants if you eventually want to replace the removable partial denture with implants.

Frequent replacement/repair. Removable partial dentures need to be replaced more frequently than bridges because the materials used to make removable partial dentures are not as resilient as materials used for bridges.

Despite the negative aspects of choosing to have a removable partial denture, there are plenty of excellent reasons why a removable partial denture might be the best choice.

Takeaway

Removable partial dentures are a great, less expensive, short-term choice for replacing missing teeth. However, most other more expensive treatments like fixed bridges and dental implants usually provide better long-term results.

Six

Root Canals

The goal of root canal treatment is to allow you to keep your natural teeth when the living part inside of the tooth must be removed. Root canal treatment is also known as *endodontic treatment.*

Root canals are done by either general dentists or by root canal specialists who are called endodontists. Dental school takes four years. Becoming a specialist in root canals takes an additional two to three years of advanced specialty dental education in endodontics. Those extra two to three years can make a big difference in an endodontist's knowledge and skill at handling difficult root canals, molar root canals, and retreating failed root canals.

The living part in the center of the tooth is called the pulp. It is composed of nerves and blood vessels. When the pulp becomes infected with bacteria or fully dies, it must be removed. When performing a root canal, the dentist takes out the pulp from the center of the tooth and also removes the nerves and blood vessels from the canal in the center of the roots. Root canals can be done to relieve pain and to stop any bacteria or dead pulp material from leaking out the tips of the canal into adjacent bone.

Another reason why a dentist may need to do a root canal is if the dentist needs to encroach upon the pulpal area to make a crown on the tooth. This is an infrequent procedure, but necessary at times. It might be needed if there was a missing tooth and the tooth in the opposite arch erupted into the empty space. The extra erupted height beyond normal needs to be trimmed down to make the new crown line up with its previous position. This extra trimming can get too close to the nerve, so a root canal is done to avoid nerve pain.

Doing a root canal relieves pain, allows you to keep teeth, and helps keep your bone height around the tooth. Root canals are extremely successful with a success rate of over 90%. And they are mandatory to keep some teeth.

If you have tooth pain, do not wait until it is so bad you need to go to an emergency room in the middle of the night. There are three reasons to go to a dentist at the earliest discomfort:

1. Root canal associated infections can be deadly.

2. Emergency room treatment by physicians often do not result in the appropriate diagnosis, treatment, or medication choices, and you still may need an extraction or root canal.

3. Emergency room visits for a painful tooth cost around $6,000.00 and a root canal can cost only $1,000.00.

The first step in performing a root canal is opening the top of the tooth. The pulp tissue and blood vessels are then removed from the center of the roots with round toothpick-shaped metal files. Sequentially larger-diameter files are used one after the other to remove all the infected pulp tissue. Some medicated solutions are used to help dissolve and clean out the tissue in the canals. Finally, a rubber-like material, called gutta-percha, is cemented into the cleaned canal space down the center canal of the roots to the end at the root tips.

Figure 6.1 is a simple depiction of where healthy nerves and blood vessels exist down the center of the tooth root.

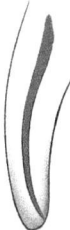

Figure 6.1. A nerve exists in the center of a tooth root.

Risks and Concerns

A root canal is often the only way to keep a tooth. However, you should be aware of some negative aspects of having a root canal done to avoid surprises. Additionally, being knowledgeable can help you keep your tooth after a root canal is performed.

Brittleness

When dentists do a root canal, they remove almost all the blood supply in the center of the tooth. Because the blood supply of the tooth has been removed, the tooth becomes brittle and dry over a period of years.

The main reason root canals fail is that the tooth has become so brittle it snaps like a dry twig. Placing a crown on a tooth that had root canal therapy performed helps reduce the risk of localized snapping forces and delays the eventual fracture of the tooth due to brittleness. You usually will need a crown placed immediately after a root canal to protect the weakened tooth.

A weaker tooth

The shape of the nerves and blood vessels inside the root are not perfectly round. The nerves and blood supply are often thin and ribbon shaped. Your dentist needs to create a round hole because round rotating instruments are used to remove all the nerve tissue and blood supply from the center of the tooth. The tooth is hollowed out all the way to the root tip during this process.

The hollowing out of the tooth reduces its structural integrity and strength by a small amount. The materials used to fill the hole created by the root canal process do not add any structural strength to the tooth. This weakened tooth has an increased risk of fracture. However, a slightly weaker tooth is almost always better than not having a tooth.

Figure 6.2 is a diagram of a cross section of a tooth. This is an extreme example to emphasize the amount of tooth removed by the rounded instruments used to extract the ribbon-shaped pulp tissue in the center of a tooth. The circle shows an exaggerated amount of tooth material removed but makes it easy to understand why a tooth could be weakened after this procedure.

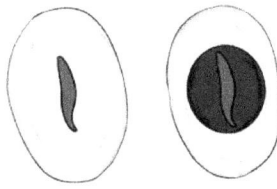

Figure 6.2. Removing the nerve hollows out the tooth.

Incomplete cleansing

It is impossible to remove or "clean out" all the living tissue inside a root since there are hundreds of tiny blood and nerve branches off the main central pulp. These branches of tissue extend from the center of the tooth to the edge of the root in contact with the jawbone. These tiny branches are cut off from their central blood supply and die during a root canal. This allows for tiny areas of dead tissue to leak into the jawbone.

Most of the time the small onslaught of dead tissue and bacteria appears to be tolerated by our bodies. The tooth will feel comfortable for many years and look healthy in an x-ray. In rare instances, the localized immune response is overwhelmed by the tiny amount of dead tissue. As a result, this immune response will destroy bone next to the leaking canals. Dentists can diagnose this bone loss from an x-ray. This missing bone means the tooth is not attached to the root and can result in root canals needing to be redone or possible tooth loss.

There is also a less common viewpoint that this interaction between your immune system and even a small amount of dead tissue and bacteria can possibly cause systemic problems not limited to the tissue adjacent to the tooth.

An instrument can break off

An instrument can break off in the center of the tooth during the root canal procedure and can lead to a failed root canal. Occasionally, leaving the broken instrument tip in the center of the tooth can result in a good long-term result, but it is best to jiggle the broken tip out if possible.

Why Root Canals Fail

Root canals done by a skilled dentist or endodontist have high success rates. But root canals *do* fail. Knowing why the procedure might fail should add important knowledge to help you make sensible dental health choices. The main causes of root canal failures are listed below.

- *The seal (obturation) at the tip of the root canal is inadequate* and leaks bacteria and dead tissue into the bone. New microorganisms can reinfect the canal system.

- *The placement of the filling material (gutta-percha or cement) in the canal extends beyond the root tip.* This is a common imperfection that usually causes no trouble, but it can result in short-term or long-term discomfort and bone loss.

- *The filling material (gutta-percha or cement) placement in the canal was not extended to the natural tip of the pulp tissue (near the tip of the root).* This allows residual dead tissue and bacteria to leak into the bone.

- *A hole was created through the side of the tooth* accidentally during the root canal procedure.

- *Existing periodontal disease on the side of the tooth* can interact with the root canal nerves and blood vessel branches and together can cause so much bone loss that the tooth needs to be extracted.

- *An adjacent tooth has pulp or periodontal disease* and that infection spreads through the bone to the root canal treated tooth.

- *The tooth is split or cracked* before, during, or after treatment.

- *The tooth fractures because it gets brittle over time.* A root canal removes the blood supply and moisture from the center of the tooth. Even under the best of circumstances, this increasing brittleness often leads to fracture after several years.

- *Trauma to the tooth* occurs resulting in fracture.

- *The dentist can miss cleaning out a main canal.* There are often more main nerve canals than there are roots. For instance, there are two main canals on the front outside root of the upper first molar over

93% of the time. One of these two canals is notoriously overlooked by dentists. Not treating the extra canal initially often causes the need for an additional subsequent root canal treatment or tooth loss. If a main canal is missed, the bone around the tooth will not heal, and the root canal needs to be redone.

- *Loss due to zipping.* If tissues are left in the canal at the root tip, dead material leaks into the bone that supports the tooth. This can lead to tooth loss. As a root canal is performed, the initial thin round files can easily curve with the curvature of the canal in the center of the root. Thicker and thicker files are needed to create a clean round hole to remove the remaining sides of the ribbon-shaped canal tissue. Thicker round wires are harder to bend than thin round wires. When thicker files do not curve with the natural shape of the pulp canal, an inadequate removal of the nerve and blood vessel tissues results. This failure of the files to curve allowing dead tissue to remain at the end of the root is called root canal zipping. Root canal zipping creates a hole at the end of the tooth that is straighter than the actual curve of the canal. (See Figure 6.3.) An inadequately cleansed area of tissue remains in the curved area adjacent to the hole. Unfortunately, failure to heal can result.

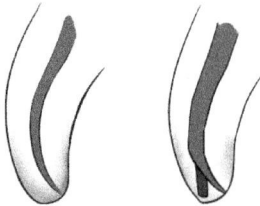

Figure 6.3. Root canal zipping.

This residual infected material in the curved canal is often not visible on the x-ray because the cement and root canal gutta-percha material block the viewing of this area. The remaining tissue leaking into the adjacent bone can cause the failure of the root canal and tooth loss.

Re-treatment

The objective of root canal therapy is to remove the infected pulp canal material from the center of the tooth. That space is then filled with a round toothpick shaped rubber-like gutta-percha and glued in place with cement. In an ideal world, this stops any remaining dead pulp tissue and bacteria from leaking out of the tooth into the jawbone. If there is leakage from these tissues and bacteria, the root canal fails. As discussed above, root canals can also fail for other reasons. If a root canal fails, the tooth needs to be extracted or treated with a new root canal procedure. This could be a new root canal through the crown of the tooth, or a different procedure called an apicoectomy.

Apicoectomy

Occasionally one of the reasons root canals fail is that a tooth root tip has too many tiny branches of the nerve and blood vessels to be completely cleaned out and sealed by the root canal procedure. In this situation, the leakage of trapped bacteria and dead tissue into the jawbone can be too much for a person's body to tolerate. This situation usually cannot be determined in advance. If the tooth with excessive branches has a failed root canal, it is possible to go in through the bone on the side of the tooth root and cut off the tip of the root higher up on the tooth (above the area of numerous branches) and seal up the main nerve and vessel canal. This procedure is an apicoectomy.

Statistics indicate an approximate 69% success rate for most conventionally retreated teeth or apicoectomy retreated teeth (success is defined as the tooth lasting for several years). This is a much lower chance of success than the success rate of more than 90% for first-attempt root canals. Re-treatment is likely to have a better success rate if done by an endodontist, a specialist in root canals, since much of their additional training involves saving teeth with initially failed root canals.

If an apicoectomy fails, you usually need to have the tooth extracted.

Apicoectomy is also performed on children, as is a procedure called apexification. Apexification is possible on teeth that are still developing or sometimes on teeth with roots that have eroded or "resorbed." In this process, the root canal of a tooth with an open apex (the end of a root) is filled with calcium hydroxide or mineral trioxide aggregate to form a calcium barrier on a tooth with a dead pulp. This process has a success rate of over 80% in children.

The Newest Research

Root canals are often mandatory, but there are plenty of less-than-ideal aspects about root canals and their longevity. Some excellent researchers have just published a retrospective study delineating a technique using a calcium silicate-based bioactive ceramic. This product may possibly eliminate the need for hollowing out the root nerve canals and the resultant discomfort and brittleness issue. Maybe further research on this topic will reveal that just removing and medicating the main chamber of the pulp will be adequate and reduce many of the negative aspects of root canals.

Takeaway

Teeth always become more brittle after root canals. You can increase your tooth longevity by remembering this and making sure not to challenge these teeth by biting or pulling on hard substances like beef jerky or opening bottles with your teeth. If the tooth eventually does crack, the next chapter deals with this unfortunate situation.

Seven

Extractions – Removing Teeth

An extraction (removing a tooth) is normally done with local anesthesia and is a type of oral surgery. Sedating the patient with drugs is occasionally required for patient comfort.

Reasons for Extractions

There are many reasons to have teeth extracted. Some of these are listed here:

- A tooth is causing persistent pain.
- Advanced periodontal disease.
- A tooth is too broken down to support a filling or crown.
- To augment the treatment of periodontal disease on adjacent teeth.
- When untreatable infections affect the nerve or blood supply of the tooth.
- When an extraction can augment the speed of orthodontic treatment.
- Assistance with orthodontics. (Sometimes selective timing of extractions can minimize the need for orthodontics.)
- Prior to head and neck radiation therapy for cancer.

- When untreatable resorption of part of the tooth occurs, especially when the cause is not understood.

- Teeth are in a bad position or impacted in the bone.

- When teeth are fractured or cracked and when teeth are involved with a jawbone fracture.

- When an extraction will help with proper alignment of restorations.

- On rare occasions you can have a condition where extra teeth erupt and create a crowding situation or teeth exhibit problems with their size, shape, or location.

- When there is infection around a wisdom tooth.

- Wisdom tooth removal (see below).

A Note about Wisdom Teeth Removal

There are some situations where wisdom teeth can play a role in causing crowding and crooked teeth, but usually wisdom teeth are only one of many factors that can cause dental crowding. If you have a choice about when to remove a wisdom tooth, it is better to take teeth out when you are younger. Younger patients heal faster than older patients. Young bone is flexible, so less trauma occurs when removing teeth. Additionally, the roots of teeth are often shorter and not fully developed in teenagers, resulting in less trauma upon removal. If wisdom teeth removal is necessary, having the teeth removed before age seventeen is ideal.

Complications

Complications can arise with any treatment. This is particularly true with extractions. Sometimes these complications are surprising and upsetting to the patient. Some complications, such as bleeding, will occur more frequently, while some rarely occur. I have included a discussion of most of these situations below. My purpose is to minimize patient anxiety about unforeseen problems that may pop up, since most resolve quickly and easily.

Bleeding

Most people do not know when bleeding becomes a serious concern. A little blood is usually expected after extractions and not of much consequence. Deciding when to get care for bleeding should be made by a call or visit to your surgeon. The Red Cross defines life-threatening bleeding based on volume and flow. If an adult loses one-half the volume of a soda can, the loss can be life threatening and immediate care is needed. This is also true if a child loses one-third of a soda can of blood. Spurting or continuously flowing blood can also become life threatening. If you are faced with either of these situations, call 911 for emergency care. Causes of bleeding are elaborated below.

- Bleeding, bruising, and swelling can result from *surgical trauma*.

- Medical conditions like *hemophilia* can result in excess bleeding.

- Bleeding can also result from taking prescription and some over-the-counter nonprescription medications as well as from drinking alcohol. Medications notorious for causing intraoperative and postoperative bleeding include those that follow. (*Brand names are capitalized, but not generic names.*)

• Coumadin	• Clopidogrel
• warfarin	• Advil
• Xarelto	• Motrin
• Rivaroxaban	• ibuprofen
• Eliquis	• Numerous others
• Apixaban	• dabigatran etexilate
• Pradaxa	• aspirin
• Plavix	

Herbal supplements that can cause bleeding include these:

- gingko biloba
- fish oil
- feverfew

- dong quai
- ginseng
- garlic

Additional herbal supplements are also suspected causes of increased bleeding and bruising. All medications that you take should be discussed with your surgeon well before the planned surgery date.

Pain

There is usually some pain after extractions, which should rapidly diminish after the fourth day following the surgery. If it does not, or gets worse, call your doctor.

Pain can be reduced by taking pain medication after the surgery is completed. It is in your best interest to take your prescribed pain medication before you feel pain to reduce the pain intensity and duration. Studies show that once you are experiencing pain there are physical changes in the nerve channels that make pain more intense and last longer.

Taking pain medications prior to surgery can increase bleeding during surgery. Consult your surgeon before taking medications prior to a procedure.

Many double-blind studies show alternating ibuprofen with acetaminophen every three to four hours will relieve pain just as well as some dangerously addictive prescription medications. Acetaminophen is found in lots of over-the-counter liquids and pills so make sure to avoid taking more than the recommended dose.

Nerve damage

Nerve damage can occur by pressing, crushing, or cutting nerves during surgery. The sensation after nerve damage can leave you with symptoms ranging from occasional discomfort to complete numbness. These symptoms can be very annoying, but they will usually go away over several weeks to months.

Hole in the sinus

Mouth-to-sinus communication (oral-antral communication) occurs when a hole develops between a sinus and your mouth. This happens most often after an upper back tooth is removed and the root tip pulls tissue out of the sinus. This causes discomfort and can cause some fluid to go from your mouth up into your nose and sinus when swallowing.

Most of the time these holes heal on their own over a few weeks to a few months. A surgical procedure can be done to slide adjacent mouth tissue over the hole if it does not heal. If your surgeon is worried this situation may exist, they may prescribe antihistamines, warn you not to blow your nose, and tell you to sneeze with your mouth open if you need to sneeze.

Dying bone

Osteonecrosis (bone inflammation and bone death) can occur in rare circumstances after extractions due to trauma or infection. Osteonecrosis can also be due to a history of a patient taking bisphosphonates and other drugs used to prevent loss of bone density. (See "The Effect of Bisphosphonate Drugs on Extractions" at the end of this chapter for a more complete explanation.)

Some drugs that can cause osteonecrosis (many are bisphosphonates) are listed below:

- Actonel (risedronate sodium)
- Atelvia (risedronate sodium)
- Benefos (clodronate sodium)
- Boniva (ibandronate sodium)
- Didronel (ibandronate sodium)
- Etidronate (Etidronate)
- Fosamax (alendronate sodium)
- Fosamax plus D (alendronate sodium/cholecalciferol)
- generic alendronate (alendronate sodium)
- Skelid (tiludronate disodium)
- Aredia (Pamidronate disodium)
- Bonefos (Clodronate disodium)
- Boniva IV (ibandronate sodium)
- Prolia (Denosumab)
- X Genia (Denosumab)
- Reclast (zoledronic acid)
- Zometa (zoledronic acid)
- Other drugs are also implicated.

Pieces of bone

Small pieces of dead bone coming out of the surgical site (osseous sequestrum) is relatively common and there is sometimes no obvious cause. This may occur because oxygen fails to be delivered to every area of bone when tiny blood vessels are inadvertently damaged during surgery. This results in small pieces of bone dying and being ejected by the body. Even if these pieces of bone can be sharp and irritating, it is usually best to allow these to come out on their own rather than removing them surgically.

Gum tissue dying

Gum tissue necrosis (dying tissue) can occur after surgery. Tissue will die from excessive crushing pressure with instruments, infection, or not maintaining a good blood supply. It is prudent for your dentist to retain a wide base when pushing the gum away from the bone for the tissue to maintain a good blood supply. If the gum is being pushed back away from the bone, the width of the gum tissue near the teeth must be narrower than the width of the tissue remaining attached to the rest of the mouth tissue. This is because blood vessels do not run perfectly parallel to the length of a tooth; some may come in from the side. On occasion the tissues cannot tolerate surgical manipulation because they are unpredictably delicate, resulting in tissue death despite proper care.

Bone infection

Osteomyelitis is a serious bone infection, and the cause is often not determinable. It is often linked to drug abuse, alcohol abuse, diabetes, or poor oral hygiene.

Damage to adjacent teeth

Damage to adjacent teeth can be minimized by careful surgical techniques.

Muscle spasm

Lockjaw/muscle spasm, also called trismus, can occur when the lower jaw is held open wider or longer during a procedure than the patient's body can accommodate.

Dry socket

Dry socket, also called *alveolar osteitis,* is a complication occurring after extractions. It is characterized by a radiating pain occurring three days or more after the surgery. Usually, the blood clot in the socket of the extracted tooth never formed or was dislodged. Food or debris is seen in the hole (socket) where the tooth was removed. A bad smell is usually present. Patients with poor oral hygiene, smokers, patients on birth control, and patients with diabetes are more likely to get a dry socket.

Your dentist will usually effectively treat a dry socket by rinsing out the socket with saline water or an antibacterial rinse and placing a paste, gauze, or other medicament in the tooth socket. Antibiotics are almost never needed.

Infections

Infections can occur with any surgery. The mouth is one of the most bacteria-ridden locations in the body and cannot be sterilized. Fortunately, the mouth is surrounded with a heavy concentration of lymph tissue. Lymph tissue makes our body's white blood cells. These white blood cells respond rapidly to the presence of bacteria, viruses, and foreign bodies in our mouth tissues and are mobilized to attack these challenges. Antibiotics are occasionally needed if infection develops despite our localized immune system's help.

Broken jaw

A broken jaw can happen during tooth removal. Areas of bone in the jaw can be weaker than ideal due to tooth loss, dental implants, previous injury, or defect. Even if the jaw is healthy and normal, excessive pressure can occasionally cause a broken jaw.

Obstructive sleep apnea

Obstructive sleep apnea can be created or magnified if the upper or lower arch length is shortened. When teeth are extracted, the extraction site space shrinks if the extraction site dimensions are not preserved with a bone graft, implant, or dental appliance. This causes the total space within the mouth to shrink in size. As a result, the tongue has less available space and is more likely to be pressed back or fall back into the throat when you sleep, potentially leading to obstructive sleep apnea and all the associated negative health ramifications. This is one reason why the recommendation to remove all wisdom teeth is decreasing and why the removal of four pre-molars to speed up orthodontics is falling out of favor.

Brain abscess

Brain abscess or cavernous sinus thrombosis can occur in extremely rare circumstances. The veins around the eye and in the face often lack the one-way valves that are present in veins elsewhere in the body. This allows blood-borne infections to pass backwards into the veins and upward to the brain. Infections in the upper jawbone are particularly dangerous because of this lack of one-way valves in the blood vessels in this area. A brain abscess can occur if you delay extractions of infected teeth.

Osteoradionecrosis

Individuals who have had radiation therapy can have osteoradionecrosis (bone death in the area of radiation therapy) after an extraction. Radiation therapy for cancer can damage the blood supply in the irradiated area. The lack of a good blood supply can limit proper healing and cause bone and tissue death after oral surgery.

Medical Conditions to Worry about Before Having Extractions

If any of the following apply to you, special precautions should be taken before extractions, or oral surgery should be avoided:

- Heart attack less than three months ago.
- Angina that is not controlled.
- Newly diagnosed heart disease.
- Recent surgery.
- Medical condition that has worsened recently.

- Stroke in the last three months.

- Placement of heart stents in the last six months.

- Recent TIAs (transient ischemic attacks).

- Not keeping up with regularly scheduled dialysis.

- Heart valve dysfunction.

- Acute respiratory distress.

There are other conditions not listed above that can also affect your decision. You must determine with your dental surgeon and your physician if your specific situation allows you to have surgery.

Pre-medication with Antibiotics

If you have certain conditions, medical complications can occur if you do not take antibiotics prior to extractions. These include having had heart valve repair or replacement with a prosthetic valve; a heart infection called endocarditis; certain types of heart disease since birth; a heart transplant for heart myopathy; and some rarer problems.

Prosthetic joints used to be included on the list of "antibiotic prophylaxis needed"; however, antibiotics are often *not* needed unless you have developed complications with your joints. Research shows there is often more risk in taking antibiotics (allergic reactions, etc.) than the risk of bacteria damaging a prosthetic joint attachment to bone in most situations.

You do not want to take antibiotics if they are not needed because, in addition to other concerns, some antibiotics can weaken the walls of arteries and cause deadly ruptures or tears in your arteries. Check with your physician about your specific issues.

Takeaway

You must discuss with your dental surgeon and your physician if your specific situation requires you to have antibiotic premedication. *It is dangerous to take antibiotics without a very good reason.*

The Effect of Bisphosphonate
Drugs on Extractions

Every bone in your body is slowly and continually remodeled throughout your life. Almost all calcium in our bodies is stored in bones. Calcium is used to help muscles and nerves work. If you are deficient of calcium in some part of your body, or need to supply calcium to a developing fetus, you can get calcium from your bones. Bone can be broken down and dissolved (resorbed) into tiny components. This dissolution of bone releases calcium. The bloodstream can then carry calcium to where it is needed most. This resorption and replacement of bone allows you to adjust for calcium needs and for microscopic and large bone repairs. In fact, all the bone in your body is resorbed and replaced at least once every ten years. There are two main types of cells associated with this bone remodeling: OsteoClasts (bone resorption cells) and OsteoBlasts (bone formation cells).

Bisphosphonates are prescribed for those with osteoporosis/osteopenia. Bisphosphonates damage and kill OsteoClasts, but do not bother OsteoBlasts. The net effect is less bone resorption but normal bone formation. This leaves you with more total bone, more dense bone, and less risk of fracture of the hip or other bones. A reduced risk of hip fracture is incredibly important. Older people with a hip fracture have a 500% to 800% increased risk of dying in the three months following the hip fracture. (Haentjens P, et al. Ann Intern Med 2010; 152:380-90).

Osteoporosis and osteopenia medications affect extraction-site healing. Medications taken to treat osteoporosis and osteopenia can cause localized bone death at the site of tooth removal. Dissolving traumatized bone and rebuilding healthy bone is how we heal after removing teeth. The interruption of the natural removal and replacement of bone by bisphosphonates and other osteoporosis and osteopenia drugs can cause trouble with tooth extraction site healing.

Sometimes your physician can allow you to take a two-month holiday from these medications before extractions and reduce your risk of poor healing and localized bone death (osteonecrosis). Using antibiotics and antimicrobials before procedures may also help reduce the risk of osteonecrosis.

Takeaway

Most patients who have a history of bisphosphonate use do well after a tooth extraction. It must be acknowledged and recognized, however, that bisphosphonates do add additional risk of complications.

Eight

Dental Implants, Part I

Implants Have Revolutionized Dentistry, but. . .

Implants replace missing teeth that in the past would have been replaced by complete dentures, removable partial dentures, or bridges. Despite being an excellent therapy, there are numerous situations where dental implants may not be as good as other treatment choices. To make the right personal choice, it is important to understand and be prepared for the negative aspects of dental implants as well as the positive aspects.

Older research, often paid for by dental implant manufacturers, supported doing dental implants in almost every situation possible. Recent research done by universities and dental scientists is revealing the disappointing truth about implant failures and showing that complications occur approximately 40% of the time.

This chapter and the next two will provide you with the knowledge of what to expect when getting implants. This information will help you chose the best option for yourself and avoid an ugly result.

What is a Dental Implant?

Dental implants consist of three main pieces (see Figures 8.1, 8.2, and 8.3):

- *Implant*: The implant is screwed into the bone where a tooth is missing.

- *Abutment:* An abutment is screwed into the implant.

- *Crown*: The crown is glued (cemented) or screwed onto the abutment.

The implant looks like a screw and is screwed into the bone replacing a missing tooth. The abutment extends from the top of the implant to above the gums. The crown is the part that slides over the abutment and looks like a tooth when you smile.

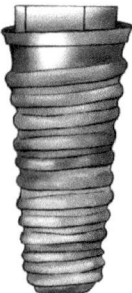

Figure 8.1. Dental implant (also called implant fixture or implant body).

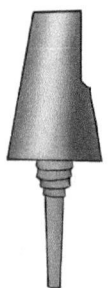

Figure 8.2. Abutment.

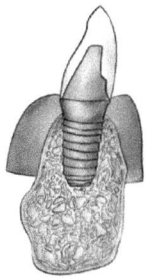

Figure 8.3. Cross section of a crown on an abutment attached to a dental implant in the jawbone.

Dental Implant Placement

The first step of replacing a tooth with an implant is to place the implant in the bone where a tooth is missing. This can be done as either a one-stage procedure or a two-stage procedure.

In a one-stage procedure, the abutment and crown are placed on the implant immediately after placing the implant into the bone. The long-term success rate of the one-stage procedure is likely to be slightly worse than the success rate of the two-stage procedure. The upside is that the one-stage procedure allows you to have your final crown sooner, but this is particularly risky in front teeth where the implant is placed immediately in the socket at the time of tooth removal. Front teeth naturally have very little bone over the front of their roots and immediate placement of the implant where the tooth was removed results in bone loss and ugly gum recession over fifty percent of the time. Extracting a front tooth and placing a bone graft in the socket, then returning in four months to place the implant in a location with more bone on the front side is likely to provide a much prettier long-term result.

During a two-stage procedure, the implant is placed in the bone on the day of surgery and covered up by the gums. After leaving the implant undisturbed for three to four months to heal and attach to the bone, the implant can be uncovered. The abutment can then be screwed into the implant and the crown glued (cemented) or screwed onto the abutment. The two-stage procedure is preferred for most candidates if long-term success is the most important consideration.

The decision to do a one-stage or two-stage procedure is based on how likely the bone will attach to the implant during healing. If you have soft bone, are a smoker, or wear a removable partial denture, it is often best to fully bury the implant under the gums and then place the abutment and crown three or four months later. This two-stage procedure is also preferred if you are a diabetic or have other health issues that make you a poorer candidate for implants.

If the dentist suggests the two-stage procedure, it is unwise to press the dentist to do the one-stage procedure because you want the crown sooner. There are many situations where a two-stage procedure is likely to give you better implant longevity. Sometimes this decision is based on clinical impression, not just on an easily explained fact or two.

Implants Serve Multiple Purposes

Implants can be used two ways: to permanently hold crowns or to allow support for removable teeth.

A crown can be permanently glued (cemented) or screwed on to the abutment/implant. These are called fixed restorations. Alternatively, the abutment/implant can be used as support for removable dental prostheses such as dentures or removable partial dentures. These dentures or partial dentures can be slid on and off a short, smooth abutment which provides vertical support and prevents them from sliding up, right, or left while chewing. These are referred to as removable implant prosthetics.

In situations where you are replacing only one or two teeth, fixed dental implants with crowns are usually a better choice than a bridge. Here's why:

- *You do not have to trim down adjacent teeth if you do a single implant.* Making a bridge requires trimming down (prepping) the teeth on either side of the missing tooth to make room to glue on the bridge. Trimming down the adjacent teeth weakens and damages those teeth. The trauma of trimming down the teeth can lead to root canals and occasionally eventual tooth loss (as explained in the chapter on root canals). If those teeth are in perfect condition, then trimming down teeth to make a bridge is often particularly unwise.

- *Bridges stress the teeth that the bridge is cemented to.* As discussed in the chapter on bridges, the teeth that the bridge is glued to must handle their own original biting forces plus the forces placed on the fake tooth (called a pontic) spanning the area where the missing tooth was. These extra forces on a bridge can jeopardize the health of the teeth where the bridge is glued. Occasionally this is too much chewing force for the teeth supporting the bridge to handle. They can fracture, the cement can break loose, or gum disease can be magnified on the teeth the bridge is cemented upon.

- *A dental implant, on the other hand, can independently handle biting forces.* A dental implant replacing one tooth independently handles the forces of chewing on that one tooth. Implants are often the best choice to replace teeth because the dental implant is placed directly where the missing teeth were.

Bear in mind this caveat: You may also consider cost in your decision. The cost of two crowns on natural teeth plus an implant with crown on it in the middle is more than the cost of a bridge. If the teeth that are going to support the bridge are already compromised and need crowns, then doing an implant is not necessarily the clear choice. This is because the supporting teeth need to be trimmed down for crowns anyway, and a bridge may be an appropriate choice rather than an implant. Trimming down a tooth for a crown is the same amount of trauma and cost as trimming down a tooth for a bridge.

Takeaways

Placing a dental implant is often an excellent choice to replace a missing tooth or teeth. The choice of placing an implant is particularly advantageous if the teeth on either side of the missing teeth are in excellent health. Another superb use of dental implants is to place two to five implants to stabilize lower full dentures. The choice to have an implant placed as a one-or two-stage procedure depends on your health, habits, impatience, bone density and your dentist's clinical impression.

Nine

Dental Implants, Part II

Are You a Candidate for a Successful Implant?

This chapter will tell you about the important factors you should consider before choosing dental implants. For instance, if you smoke more than ten cigarettes a day, your implants may rapidly fail. Taking the time to review all the factors that may affect your success is important. Your dentist can determine if you have enough bone in the right place for dental implants and decide if they feel you are technically a good candidate for dental implants. Unfortunately, your dentist's determination can be incomplete because it does not include all the complex combination of factors that often only you know about yourself.

Your dentist might not get all the critical information from you due to limitations on the length of the health history and time spent in conversation with the dentist. I have never seen a patient over age thirty-five who had included *all* important aspects that can affect implants on the health history forms they filled out. Only a long discussion brings extra issues to light. Even with a long discussion, many concepts important to your success are often overlooked.

Your dentist can use general statistics to establish the value of doing implants. A general statement often heard in a dental office is 90% of dental implants last ten years or longer. This may be true under certain circumstances, but you are unlikely to be exactly the average patient. In fact, the 90% rule is beginning to be questioned in many situations.

Your Personal Assessment

Once a dentist says you can have implants placed, you need to consider your own personal factors as well.

Are you the kind of person, for example, who will practice excellent oral hygiene around the implant and without fail go every three months to the hygienist for implant and periodontal maintenance? If you don't feel like you can commit to this kind of effort, your implant can be lost as much as five times faster than a natural tooth already compromised with periodontal disease.

You also need to consider your unique health history, including drug and alcohol use, smoking, and your family health history, rather than relying completely on your dentist to decide if you are a good candidate for implants.

You can become a smart consumer of dental care. Every patient has a very different set of health conditions that must be considered when deciding whether to do implants. It is in your best interest to determine whether your complex set of conditions will result in an implant longevity that will meet your expectations.

The Clinical Factors

Aside from assessing your personal health and resolve, you need to understand the key clinical factors your dentist will be concerned with before you commit to this surgical procedure. Some of these concepts are described below.

Are you medically fit?

A careful analysis of your medical fitness to tolerate the surgery to place dental implants needs to be made beforehand. Some implantologists use the American Society of Anesthesiologists health evaluation to determine whether a patient is fit enough to undergo dental implant surgery. This analysis is independent of, and should come before, a discussion of whether the implant, when completed, will attach to the bone and the likelihood of its long-term success.

Classification ASA I is a normal healthy person who does not smoke and consumes minimal alcohol. ASA II is a patient with one mild disease only and may be a smoker or social alcohol drinker and have well-controlled blood pressure or diabetes. Patients who fall into ASA I and ASA II classifications tolerate dental implant surgery well in most situations.

Classification ASA III includes patients with one or more moderate to severe diseases and certain risk factors, including cardiovascular problems, high blood pressure, poorly controlled diabetes, morbid obesity, COPD, heavy alcohol use, active hepatitis, and undergoing current dialysis. These patients do not do as well during dental implant surgery and should make sure they are going to have an experienced dentist and physician team monitoring their health.

Reasons to consider avoiding implants

If you have had any of the following, you should get a careful analysis of these issues before considering any dental implant surgery.

- Recent heart attack or stroke.

- Heart valve prosthesis surgery.

- Immunosuppression due to a disease process or drug induced.

- Active treatment for cancer.

- Drug abuse.

- Bone disease or taking medication for bone cancer.

- Head and neck radiation therapy, even in the distant past.

- Osteopenia/osteoporosis and associated medications. Osteopenia is a condition of low bone density. Osteoporosis is more severe and may weaken the bone and put you at even greater risk for fractures. Implants rely on attaching to bone. If there is less bone to hold onto, the implant is not as solidly attached. Patients with osteopenia or osteoporosis may have a poorer implant prognosis since the implant is placed in less dense bone. The good news is that excellent results can usually still be attained despite having these conditions. More importantly, perhaps, are how the effects of the medications taken for osteopenia or osteoporosis can affect your dental implant success.

- Bisphosphonate use (especially intravenous). If you have taken intravenous bisphosphonates, instead of just pills, you are more likely to have a problem with dental implants (and possibly with extractions also). If you have taken only oral bisphosphonates (not intravenous), this risk is reduced but still present. An analysis of your dosage, type of administration, and how long you have been taking bisphosphonates can help determine the risk of implant failure.

- Some drugs other than bisphosphonates also pose implant failure risk. Make sure you tell your dentist if you have been treated for bone cancer, osteoporosis, or osteopenia.

A1C diabetes test results

Uncontrolled diabetes significantly reduces dental implant success. High blood sugar levels inhibit healing and increase infection risk due to reduced immune system function.

The amount of bone

Bone on the cheek side of an implant needs to be at least 2 mm thick to achieve a decent appearance over the long-term. If the bone on the cheek side is very thin, the bone and gum eventually just dissolve away (resorbs) and reveals the implant. Most dental implants are grey in color and can be ugly if they are visible. The dentist should be concerned if the bone on the cheek side of the implant is less than 2 mm thick. Sometimes a slice of the root on the cheek side can be left attached to the bone and retained (socket shield procedure) to protect the tissue from receding.

The amount of dense, attached gum tissue

It is important to have enough dense, attached gum tissue 360 degrees around an implant to protect the bone and reduce recession. Having only loose, moveable cheek tissue around an implant rather than having 2 to 3 mm of dense attached gum tissue can lead to: gum recession; loss of bone and tissue attachment to the implant; more plaque accumulation; more gingival inflammation; bleeding upon probing; and sensitive gums when brushing your teeth.

The distance between the implant and the adjacent teeth

Having enough space around the implant is important. You need to have at least 3 mm between implants. You also need 2 mm between a natural tooth and an implant. Without these distances the bone is not likely to stay healthy.

Infections before placement

It is never good to have implants placed in an area where the bone is actively infected. The dentist will usually try to remove the infection by scraping out the infected tissue, using antibiotics, and possibly performing laser treatment in the infected area. The dentist may place a graft or let the area heal on its own. Eventually the dentist will place the implant in the area once the bone has healed.

Missing teeth

If the teeth that are being replaced have been missing for a long time, the jawbone height and width in the area have already shrunk. A dental implant needs strong bone around it to handle the stresses of chewing. A thinned-out jawbone presents serious difficulties when trying to place a dental implant. As mentioned earlier, if the implant does not have 2 mm of bone beyond the implant on both the cheek and tongue sides, the implant might be compromised. The implant also needs to be deep enough in the bone to support the part of the abutment and crown sticking out above the gums as well.

In addition, if the length of the dental implant comprises most of the entire jawbone height in the area, this can lead to jaw fracture at the time of placement or even years later. If you need to add additional bone height through bone grafting, you should realize that building back bone height is expensive and somewhat unpredictable.

Need for a surgical stent

Your dentist might suggest that you pay for a surgical stent. A surgical stent is a device to help the dentist line up the angle and position for drilling the holes for the implant, rather than lining up the holes visually. Ideally, a surgical stent helps the dentist position the exact placement of the implant in the bone, but manufacturing flaws and improper placement of the stent can add additional errors if not done correctly. Your dentist will know if a surgical stent is needed.

The brand of implant

Confirm that the implant is from a reputable company. Make sure the brand of implant is from one of the largest and best-known implant companies. Things do go wrong with implants. You want to make sure that the implant company is still around five to ten years from now because you are likely to need repairs to your implant. Many implant companies have gone bankrupt and disappeared, and the parts and pieces needed to repair these implants are no longer available. If you cannot get replacement parts, it can mean you will need to take out the old implant and hope you have enough bone to place a new one.

Each implant can cost the dentist anywhere from $90 to $700. The cheapest implants are usually from untested companies that have no long-term studies of success. A dentist might want to use these cheaper implants to attract patients with a lower fee. Getting the cheapest implant today from a company that may not be in business five years from now can cause you significant expense and frustration when you need repairs. Choose a dentist who uses a brand name implant. These are rarely the dentists who advertise an extremely low fee.

The Risks

In addition to the general questions about the procedure and the implant, you should explore with your dentist the risks associated with the implant procedure.

Peri-implantitis. At nine years, about half of all implants have significant peri-implantitis, an infection in the bone and gum around the implant. Peri-implantitis is a major cause of implant failure. Many cases of peri-implantitis can be treated and improved surgically.

Penicillin allergy. New research shows if patients are allergic to penicillin their success with dental implants is significantly reduced. The reason for this is not fully understood yet.

"Black Triangle Disease." Two dental implants placed next to each other usually lead to the loss of gum tissue height between the implants resulting in an ugly, triangular open space that traps food. Prevention and repair of this space is

difficult. If possible, it is better not to place two implants immediately adjacent to each other in the visible areas of the smile. A way to avoid creating this triangular space is by having one implant placed in one of the two missing teeth spots and replacing the second tooth with a fake tooth hanging off the implant crown.

Implants are lost much faster if you have a history with gum disease. Implants are lost much faster if you currently have untreated gum disease elsewhere in your mouth. The bacteria on your upper right do not know that they should not swim over to your new implant on your lower left.

Fixing failing dental implants is usually more expensive and involves a greater likelihood of complications than surgically salvaging natural teeth. (Nikolaos Donos et al. Periodontol 2000. 2012 Jun.) Dental insurance policies usually pay much less towards dental implants than treating natural teeth.

If you have a problem with the implant that is not detected immediately upon placement, it is easiest to remove the implant at ten days after initial placement. The longer the implant is in place after ten days, the more extra bone that may need to be removed if it fails.

The Benefits

Implants help preserve your jawbone. If you extract teeth and do not replace them with an implant or by placing a bone graft in the socket, substantial bone height and width in the area will shrink away. This bone loss is particularly significant during the first year after the extraction. Close to half of the total eventual bone loss occurs during the first year after the extraction. Implants and socket bone grafts help preserve your jawbone.

Chewing forces are transmitted to the bone via the dental implant and these forces stimulate the bone and help keep the bone from dissolving around the implants. In fact, bone loss around dental implants placed in a socket is minimal compared to the bone loss seen in spaces where teeth are removed and the socket space is not replaced by implants or bone grafts.

Cavities. Dental implants do not get cavities like natural teeth.

Implants can help denture users. Implants can be used to solidly support dentures and removable partial dentures. Implants can also provide support to dentures to hold out your lips and cheeks to prevent wrinkles.

Older age does not stop implant success. Advanced age itself is not a reason to avoid having dental implants placed.

Average implant longevity. Some researchers suggest that the average crown placed on an implant remains attractive for around five years. The average implant remains functional for around ten years. Some implants can last more than twenty years. Of course, a natural tooth can last more than eighty years.

Dental Implants Can Be Superb, but . . .

Dental implants are a great alternative to not having a tooth, but nearly every scientific analysis shows dental implants are significantly inferior to natural teeth. As mentioned above, fixing failing dental implants is usually more expensive and involves a greater likelihood of complications than surgically salvaging natural teeth.

Unlike our natural teeth, implants do not move and flex. The metal-to-bone implant attachment, for example, is inferior to a natural tooth's attachment to bone. Natural tooth roots are attached to the bone by a layer of tissue and cells called the periodontal ligament. The periodontal ligament is like a sock around a foot; teeth can move around a little bit in this sock. This periodontal ligament can act like a shock absorber on a car, allowing the tooth to comfortably flex with pressure. This living sock of cells and tissues can respond to challenges placed upon a tooth.

If you place constant pressure in the same direction on a tooth, the cells in the periodontal ligament can allow the tooth to move within the bone. This happens because the cells around the tooth root dissolve bone on the pressure side of the tooth and fill in new bone on the tooth's opposite side as it moves. This slow movement is how orthodontics can move and straighten teeth. Teeth move a little bit every day even without orthodontics. This movement is the result of changes in the strength of the muscles of the tongue, lips, cheeks, and biting forces.

Since dental implants do not have a sock of tissues around them, there are no cells to dissolve bone and move the implant in response to gentle directional pressures. Without any intervening periodontal ligament, dental implants have a direct connection between the implant and the jawbone. This is called osseointegration, which is the direct implant-to-bone attachment. The biting forces on an implant cannot be distributed all the way down the implant and spread out into the bone like a natural tooth since the long sock of periodontal ligament is missing on an implant. This means the biting forces placed on an implant are mostly concentrated at the bone to implant attachment area just under the gums, not down deep in the bone. This partly explains why bone loss that can result in implant failure (peri-implantitis) occurs on implants up near the gums, not deep in the bone. Proximity to bacteria in your mouth is another reason.

This direct attachment to the bone also means dental implants stay solidly in the bone where you place them. Dental implants are not able to be moved around once they attach to the bone. This immobility creates several unique issues which will be explained below. Complications can arise because implants permanently attach to the bone and do not behave like natural teeth.

Orthodontics must be done first. If you want to have orthodontics to straighten your teeth, you must make sure any orthodontics you want to do is done prior to the placement of implants since implants do not move with orthodontics.

Space can open up between an implant and a tooth because natural teeth move over time. As we age, teeth tend to drift forward around the curve of the arch toward the midline of our mouths (directly under our noses) because our lip muscles get weaker, our bone density reduces, and our bite muscles press teeth forward. This is often why orthodontics done to fix crooked front teeth tends to fail and teeth get misaligned again if a retainer is not used forever.

The teeth drift toward the midline but implants never move. Over time, the movement of teeth towards the midline creates a small space between the front of implants and the natural tooth that has drifted forward. This space can trap food and lead to bone loss. The spaces can occasionally become unsightly or irritating because of food impaction. The only way to correct this problem is to replace the restoration on the implant or on the adjacent tooth to restore the once tight contact.

If after considering the concerns above, you and your dentist have decided you are a good candidate for dental implants, the final information you need is whether you can accept the complications and success rate you will face. We cover this topic in the next chapter.

∽

> *You should not get implants if you are young because your jaws are still growing and teeth are erupting, but implants stay stationary.*

During normal growth between childhood and your early twenties, teeth erupt vertically into your mouth and the jawbone develops around them. The jawbone gets larger and taller with the erupting teeth until you quit growing.

If you have an implant placed before your teeth fully erupt, the jawbone that erupts with the teeth does not pull the implant up with the rest of your teeth. Since the teeth erupt and the implant stays exactly where you place it, the teeth adjacent to a dental implant will grow to be taller than the implant. Therefore, you do not want to have an implant placed before you are age twenty (or even up to age twenty-three or so in some cases).

There are four problems if an implant is placed when you are still growing:

1. Your gumline will not look natural because the gumline on the implant will not have moved in sync with the gumline on the adjacent erupting teeth. There will be a dip in the gumline where the implant never grew taller, but the adjacent teeth did.

2. The way your upper and lower teeth come together is also affected. The teeth will not bite together as there is a difference in occlusion height. The natural upper and lower teeth come together normally as they erupt. However, the implant tooth never erupts taller and stays at its shorter position. This leaves a space above the implant, so the opposing tooth does not chew against it.

3. Also, in some instances, the tooth on the opposite arch from the implant can over erupt into the space available due to the implant being shorter. This can make a jumbled bite. This can cause temporomandibular joint (TMJ) problems and/or lead to a need for orthodontics.

4. If the jawbone has continued to grow after implant placement, a new restoration may need to be placed on the implant or the opposing bite may need to be adjusted. If you must cut out an implant and redo it, you will lose a lot of bone and it is difficult and expensive to get the gumline looking perfectly natural again.

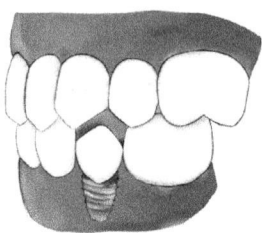

Figure 9.1. An implant does not erupt with a growing jaw.

If a dental implant is placed too early on a growing person, a gap develops when the other teeth continue to erupt and the jawbones grow taller.

Special precautions must be taken when providing implant-retained removable prosthetics for patients who suffer from dementia or memory problems.

It is common for those with dementia or memory problems to stop wearing their denture or partial denture. This can be because they do not arrange frequent appointments with their dentist to adjust the appliances so that they remain comfortable. Additionally, many people tend to be less concerned with their appearance if they develop dementia.

A serious problem occurs if those with dementia, or anyone at all, chooses not to wear their removable denture or removable partial if they are supported by implants.

When a person quits using an implant-retained removable denture or removable partial, the implant structure sticking out above the gums can damage the opposite gums, tongue, and cheeks. The implant structure above the gums should be removed and smooth caps should be placed over the implants to minimize damage to tissues. The person should then use denture adhesive for the instances in which they need to use their denture.

Regular cleaning of the implants, dental devices, and teeth is particularly important as senior adults have poorer immune systems and often experience more inflammation from plaque. Tongue bacteria can accumulate heavily, but it can be easily removed with daily use of a tongue scraper.

Bacteria associated with gum disease also pose a pneumonia risk and must be attended to with subgingival scaling and root planing. It has been shown that weekly cleaning by a dental hygienist decreases pneumonia and death risks in patients that do not brush daily.

Ten

Dental Implants, Part III

Success Rates and Complications

The success rate of dental implants for back teeth is often quoted at 91% for ten years (Nikolai J. Attard, George A. Zarb, JPD 2003). Similar statistics are quoted for implants on front teeth. Despite these rosy statistics, the reality is that these ten years are often laden with additional trips to the dentist to keep these implants functioning. These additional trips to fix a problem or remove an implant are considered *complications.*

Complication Data

Fixed implant restorations, such as implants with permanent crowns and bridges attached, have an approximately 39% complication rate over five years (Jung et al. Clin Oral Implants Res 23(Suppl 6):2-21, 2012). Removable implant prosthetics, such as a denture or partial supported by implants, have a complication rate at over 50% (Serrano et al. Rev ESp Cirug Oral Maxillofac 2006). In contrast, natural teeth have a much lower complication rate of 5% over five years.

When a patient is told there is a lower percent implant complication rate, it is usually from a study that looks at a much shorter duration. Before embarking on obtaining dental implants, the knowledgeable consumer should realize that the implant complication rate is often quoted at 13.9% from a study by McDermott (McDermott et al. Int J Oral Maxillofac Implants. Nov-Dec 2003). This study was done by excellent researchers, but the average duration of implants studied was 13.1 months. We all want and expect our expensive dental work to last significantly longer than thirteen months, so the better statistics to use are those from the two different studies by Jung and Serrano above, with an average five-year study length.

The Potential Complications

As you now know, complication rates with dental implants are high, but let's look at the specific complications to help you decide if you can accept them.

Bleeding

Post-implant bleeding can occur. Bleeding results in significant bruising around 25% of the time. The bruising can extend from the bottom of the eye, around the lips, and even down the neck onto the chest.

Bleeding is much more prevalent when you are on blood-thinning medications. You need to work with your doctor to carefully control and evaluate which blood-thinning medications and dosages are best for you. Abruptly stopping aspirin and other blood-thinning medications for a few days before the placement of the dental implant might reduce bleeding risk, but it can increase your risk of a stroke or other cerebrovascular incident 200% to 500%. An intermediate bridge medication to replace your normal blood thinner is often prescribed to reduce this additional cardiovascular risk.

A rare, but critical, complication of cutting an artery can also cause bleeding problems. The sublingual artery lies against the lower surface of the bottom jaw in a depression under the roots of the teeth. In rare instances the implant preparation hole can go too deep and penetrate the bottom of the jawbone and slice into the sublingual artery. Perforating the sublingual artery results in bleeding deep in the tissues under the tongue. This bleeding can cause a critical problem as the tissues under the tongue can swell with blood. This swollen tissue can lift the tongue and block the airways and stop the ability to breathe. There have been fatal instances of this complication. Three-dimensional x-rays such as CBCT and CAT scans prior to implant placement significantly minimize this risk.

Nerve damage

Nerves need to be avoided. These include the inferior alveolar nerve, the lingual nerve, the infra-orbital nerve, and the anterior mental loop of the inferior alveolar nerve. Damaging these structures can result in tenderness, numbness, and strange sensations.

If the placement of an implant cuts or presses on a nerve, the result can be permanent or transient pain, numbness, or both. This situation occurs much more commonly on the lower jaw. Standard dental x-rays are often not adequate for implant placement. Some studies show even panoramic x-rays do not show the exit hole of a major lower jaw nerve (mental foramen) 30% of the time. Traditional individual x-rays and panoramic x-rays also do not accurately represent distance in the jawbone. Choosing implant lengths and widths to safely avoid nerves can be misjudged using just these types of x-rays. Three-dimensional x-rays like CBCT and CAT scans can minimize this risk. Occasionally there are nerve branches not visualized even in these specialized x-rays. In rare instances unexplained numbness or discomfort can occur after dental implant placement. Luckily, nerve damage is rare.

Infections

Infections after dental implant placement occur around 1% of the time. If you have diabetes and your HA1C blood test is above nine, you are much more likely to have an infection and implant failure. When uncontrolled diabetics have bone or soft tissue grafts placed at the time of the implant, the infection rates are also much higher.

There are two lines of thought about preventing infection that apply to most patients. One option is giving two grams of amoxicillin one hour before the implant procedure and no subsequent antibiotics. Another option is to give the patient amoxicillin (500 mg) three times a day for three to four days. If the patient is diabetic, this may be extended to continue for seven days. Amoxicillin is not used for penicillin-allergic patients.

Antibiotic use in general is quite controversial now and different regimens may be used. Your dentist must evaluate your health, allergies, and the surgery to determine what is best for you.

Allergy and sensitivity

Most dental implants are made of titanium alloy. This is the same material used in hip and knee replacements. A small percentage of the population is allergic to titanium (fewer than 0.5%). The placement of the implant may be a person's first indication of this sensitivity. You can choose to have ceramic or Zirconia implants instead of titanium if you have this sensitivity.

Some practitioners promote ceramic implants because they can result in better esthetics and light transmission. Ceramic implants are white, so the grey color of metal implants does not show through thin tissue. Ceramic advocates believe tissue acceptance and biological responses to ceramic materials are better than with titanium. Despite some favorable aspects of ceramic material, ceramic implants are more fragile, crack easier, and have fewer parts and pieces available to accommodate the unique shape of your jaw.

Most dental implants continue to be made of titanium because of titanium's strength, tolerability by most people, long history of scientific success, and availability of all the parts and pieces to customize the implant to the uniqueness of each patient.

Embolism

Most dental handpieces that are used to hold the rotating burs used to trim away tooth structure and bone are air driven. To gain access to the roots and bone under the gums, the gum tissue can be pushed back (reflected) away from the bone and teeth in one sheet. The handpiece can spray air into the tissues during surgical manipulation under reflected gum tissue. It is possible to have the handpiece blow too much air into the tissues. This can result in embolism. An embolism is a blockage causing obstruction of blood and oxygen flow in a blood vessel like a blood clot or air bubble. Injuries from embolisms are extremely rare, but they can occur. Most implant dentists use rear exit air-driven handpieces so the air is not blowing directly into the tissues.

Over-tightening

If the dentist over-tightens the implant, excessive pressure on the bone can be created. Pressure on the bone can cause the bone to die and you can lose the implant. Instruments exist to provide proper pressure when placing the implant into the bone. Alternatively, if the bone is too soft to resist the proper insertion pressure and the implant just spins at the time of placement, poorer results may occur, especially if a one-stage procedure is chosen.

Soft bone issues

Implant success is better in dense bone than in bone that is less dense (soft bone). Dense bone has more bone cells to hold onto the implant initially and it takes more infection to dissolve away the bone once the implant is in function.

Bone density varies among people. Bone density varies as well in different parts of your jaw and between the upper and lower jaws. The upper jaw usually is much less dense and has poorer implant success than the lower jaw.

Despite great looking bone in x-rays, soft bone may be present. Implants can also drop or curve into a large marrow space or area of soft bone upon placement. If this happens, the implant needs to be retrieved immediately and a subsequent procedure may need to be done.

Contaminated implant

On rare occasions the implant surface is contaminated at the factory or during the procedure. This will prohibit the bone from attaching to the implant and result in failure.

Bone heated up

If the bone is heated up due to friction caused by the dental burs when creating the hole for the implant placement (surgical osteotomy), the bone cells can die and cause rapid loss of the dental implant. Using sharp new burs, ensuring proper drilling speed, and applying cooling water irrigation are standard methods to reduce the risk.

Inadequate spacing

Spacing for implants needs to be a minimum of 3 mm of bone between two implants and a minimum of 1½ to 2 mm of bone between an implant and a natural tooth. If this much space is not maintained, new bone loss and loss of gum tissue height can occur.

Sinus elevation surgery

If you need more bone to place a longer implant in the upper arch, the dentist can add bone to the bottom of the upper jawbone (maxillary) sinus. This is called sinus elevation surgery. Risks of sinus elevation surgery include sinus perforation (it happens in 10 to 30% of cases); bleeding complications due to damaging the blood supply in the bone; infections; and dizziness. Dizziness due to sinus elevation surgery is called *benign paroxysmal positional vertigo* and it occurs in 1% to 4% of these sinus surgeries. (Learn more about this topic at the end of this chapter.)

Multiple implants

You may need at least three or more implants for support if you are going to have multiple teeth replaced by a one-piece fixed or removable bridge. If implants are placed to support a long span of multiple teeth, the implants usually should be slightly staggered rather than placed in a straight line. A straight line of implants is not nearly as strong as a staggered set and can lead to fracture of all the implants or fracture of the bone supporting the implants.

Bruxism

Some people have large chewing muscles or a habit of clenching or grinding their teeth. These extra strong biting forces are one of the most common causes of implant loss during the first year or two. Clenching or grinding the teeth at night (and sometimes during the day) is called bruxism.

People who brux do not usually just grind back-and-forth over the entire mouthful of teeth; they usually tend to grind heavily on one spot. The dentist can provide a night guard to reduce the risk of this focused damage. A night guard snaps over the teeth and distributes the forces evenly on the entire biting surface so one implant or tooth does not take all the clenching and bruxing forces. Make sure you get tested for sleep apnea before wearing a night guard. Some studies show that over half of patients with sleep apnea have bruxism due to clenching their teeth at night during low oxygen events. If you have obstructive sleep apnea, wearing a night guard can block your airway and make it more difficult to breathe. Quite often a mandibular advancement device can be a better choice than a traditional night guard. Bruxism can be due to sleep disorders, emotional distress, and bite issues, or develop as a patient's habitual coping mechanism.

Gum disease

If you have a history of gum disease (periodontitis), the prognosis of an implant lasting a long time is diminished. Habits, existing bacteria, genetics, lack of cleaning your teeth well, or lack of dental visits, can increase the proportion and number of bad species of bacteria in your mouth. These bacteria can cause the bone to be destroyed around implants just like they cause bone loss around teeth. Controlling gum disease before implants are placed is mandatory.

Connecting a tooth to an implant

There are special concerns, too, if you connect an implant to a natural tooth with a bridge. An implant is immobile, but a natural tooth can move around under chewing forces. The periodontal ligament around a natural tooth allows a small amount of vertical movement with chewing. If there are excess pressures on the natural tooth, there will be bone resorption around the root tip, and the natural tooth will intrude permanently into a new position deeper in the bone. An implant that is attached to the other side of the bridge cannot move. Over time this results in the natural tooth being positioned permanently deeper into the bone and resultant loss of biting contact. This extra movement can also increase the risk of screw loosening, fracture of the implant, or fracture of the implant screw. Sometimes this situation works well for years despite these issues.

Loss of proprioception

Natural teeth have nerve endings in the layer of tissue (periodontal ligament) around the root. The nerves in this layer of tissue tell you what is going on with the tooth when you chew or press on the tooth (proprioception). The feeling you get when you bite on something hard makes you open your mouth and reduce biting force to keep you from breaking your tooth. Since implants do not have nerve endings around them, you lose this extra sensation. This makes it more difficult to stop biting when you hit something hard in your food. This failure to warn you about excess pressure can possibly lead to breaking your implant crown, implant screw, your implant, or the opposing tooth. Loss of proprioception also gives you less information about what is going on in your mouth and less aware-ness of oral movement changes than if you had natural teeth. Jaw pain and temporomandibular joint issues can be created by these excess forces.

Damage to adjacent teeth

If the bur used to make the hole for the implant is not lined up properly, the adjacent teeth can be damaged. Minor scratching of the adjacent tooth root should be recorded by the dentist and carefully watched for changes in the health of the tooth in the future. If an adjacent tooth root is drilled deeply into, however, a root canal may need to be done right away, or possibly an extraction of the tooth.

The risk of damage to the adjacent tooth can be minimized by using a sur-gical stent or taking x-rays with a metal post or drill in place where the initial narrowest hole has been drilled before completing the sequence of larger drills used to widen the hole.

Ingestion of foreign objects

It is a common complication of implant placement to drop implants, screw-drivers, crowns, and tiny screws in a patient's mouth. If a patient gags or swallows before the dentist can retrieve the item, it will end up in the lung or in the stomach. This means a trip to the emergency room for an x-ray or pos-sible surgery. A recent case occurred where an implant screwdriver ended up in a person's appendix requiring surgical removal.

If you notice the dentist has dropped something in your mouth, keep your mouth open, do not swallow, and stay calm. Teamwork by an excellent dental assistant and dentist with years of experience working together can usually retrieve it.

If you are uncomfortable during a procedure, and the dentist is on your right side, raise your left hand to catch their attention and do not talk or bump them.

Same-day crown placement on an
implant allows a quicker return to
good esthetics but poses risks.

If a crown is placed on top of the implant on the same day the implant is placed, the dentist must make sure the implant crown is not able to be hit hard by teeth on the opposite arch. Tapping on the crown can prevent the implant from becoming attached to the bone. You must avoid vigorously tapping the crown during normal chewing. Chewing force tapping can stop the direct implant-to-bone attachment (osseointegration) from occurring and lead to implant loss.

To avoid this issue, one option is placing the crown on top of the implant four months after the implant is placed in the bone. Your dentist puts the implant in the bone and covers it with gum tissue (the crown is attached a few months later). This allows you to avoid tapping on the implant while it is attaching to the bone. This is especially important if the bone is soft. After three to six months, the dentist can uncover the implant and place the crown. Another option is to make a temporary crown smaller than ideal (so that it does not get tapped on by the opposing teeth) and place it on the implant on the same day the implant is placed in the bone. Three months later the properly sized crown can be placed.

If you have specific health conditions, you may not wish to have the crown placed the same day. It is better to let the implant heal undisturbed under the gums for several months to increase the success of your dental implant.

Failures Before and After Fusion to Bone

Failure types can be defined as occurring before or after the bone has fused to the implant. Fusion to the bone starts to happen at six to twelve weeks after placement. As mentioned earlier, the binding of the bone to the implant is called osseointegration. (Osseointegration is not a true scientific term; it was chosen by a focus group in the 1980s.)

During the first few months

If the implant fails in the first few months, the most common reasons are as follows:

- **Infection.**
- **Trauma**. The surgical placement of the implant can cause more trauma than a particular person's body can tolerate. Some people can handle biologic stress better than others.
- **Chewing and biting forces** on a temporary or permanent crown placed on top of the implant are too strong and prevent the dental implant from forming a strong connection to the bone.
- **Drugs** (prescription and recreational) may cause implant failure.
- **The bone was overheated** during placement.
- **Implant rejection** which can be due to **contamination on the implant surface** from dirt, oil, microorganisms, or intolerance to the implant material.
- **The implant never got a good tight fit** into the hole that was drilled for the implant, or the **pressure used to screw the implant in was too excessive.** There is an ideal range of pressure associated with placing the implant. You do not want the implant to just spin in the hole, but you do not want the implant to be too tightly crushed against the bone upon placement.

After osseointegration

After the bone attaches to the implant, the most common causes of failure or complications are listed here:

Loosening of the screw holding the abutment or the crown. This is very common and not a complete failure since it can be fixed. A screw that has loosened can be replaced or tightened.

Complications due to breakage of the screw holding the crown. On many occasions, a broken screw can be backed out and replaced by a methodical and painstaking dentist. This is time-consuming but is a much better solution than removing the implant.

Fracture of the screw holding the abutment to the implant or **fracture of the actual implant.**

Peri-implant mucositis. This is a chronic infection by bacteria around the implant. About half of all implants develop this soft-tissue infection. When there is loose, movable gum tissue (unattached mucosa) around implants, you are more susceptible to peri-implant mucositis. Tough gum tissue called "keratinized tissue" is the ideal type of tissue to have surrounding an implant. People have genetically different amounts of keratinized tissue. In contrast to loose, movable mouth tissue like that seen inside the cheeks, keratinized tissue is often lighter pink in color and is found on the top of jawbone ridges. Keratinized attached tissue does not move when you stretch your cheek. If there is not enough heavy, strong keratinized gum tissue around the implants, the tissue to implant attachment does not resist bacteria as well as heavier tissue. It is prudent to have at least 2 mm of keratinized tissue that is strongly bound down to bone surrounding implants. It is easy for your dentist to add keratinized tissue if needed by placing a soft tissue graft. Ideally, you want to do this before or at the time of implant placement.

Peri-implantitis. Peri-implantitis is an infection causing the loss of bone supporting dental implants. Research shows this infection affects a minimum of 10% of implants and up to 43% of implants in the first several years. A normal amount of bone loss is around 1 mm in the first year and less than 0.2 mm in each of the following years. The bone loss is much more rapid in peri-implantitis. Peri-implantitis can lead to the loss of the implant and peri-implantitis repair efforts are extremely unpredictable. There is zero scientific proof that the bone actually attaches to the implant surface even if x-rays show bone grows back around an implant after repair efforts.

Improper seating. Bone loss around implants can be due to a failure to completely tighten the crown to the abutment or tighten the abutment to the implant. Sometimes bone or soft tissue can prevent the tightening needed. Care must be taken to make sure these tissues are not in the way of a proper tightening. X-rays can show when proper tightening has been achieved when the two flat surfaces are touching perfectly.

Poor oral hygiene. A dental implant is more difficult to keep clean than a natural tooth. Implant-retained crowns often have large abrupt overhangs beyond the implant edge that are hard to reach under. This is particularly true of smaller diameter implants. In addition, implants have hard to clean threads which can be colonized by bacteria in the depth of these threads and cause bone loss as they grow around the implant threads and down into the bone. A tooth root is much smoother and easier-to-clean than a threaded surface. These issues pose a problem for the patient and for the dental hygienist.

Smoking. Smoking affects the quality and quantity of blood supplied to the bone and gum tissues. Smoking also decreases the quality of the bone marrow over time.

Diabetes. Controlled diabetics do better than uncontrolled diabetics. Having a number below 8 on the A1C glucose blood test is best.

Alcohol abuse.

Periodontitis-associated bacteria spreading to the implants.

An implant that is too short can cause problems. A problem can be caused if the depth that the implant is buried in the bone is much less than the height of the crown attached to the implant and its abutment. For instance, having more than 12 mm of crown height above the top of an implant that is only 8 or 10 mm in the bone can occasionally lead to too much leveraged trauma and implant loss.

Heavy grinding or clenching beyond normal chewing activity.

Cement can prevent effective cleaning. When extra cement is left on the deep edge of the crown after it is glued to the implant, the cement makes a bulbous outcrop that sticks out from the implant surface. This protruding outcrop of cement provides the bacteria a place to hide under and avoid removal. This makes it difficult to clean the bacteria out from under the gums. Crowns can be cemented on the implant or attached to the implant with a screw. Cemented crowns can have better esthetics, especially in the front teeth. Unfortunately, it is difficult to perfectly remove any excess cement below the gum line. The alternative is to retain your crown with a screw. This allows your dentist to unscrew and replace the crown if need be. The downside is there is one more screw that can break or loosen. A complete risk analysis and comparison suggests that, if you are given a choice, screw-retained crowns are usually a better option than cemented crowns.

Use of proton pump inhibitor drugs to treat conditions like GERD can result in increased implant failure.

An Epstein Barr viral infection can increase dental implant failure rates.

Dental implants placed next to teeth with endodontic problems like infections at the root tip can fail due to local spreading of the infection from the diseased tooth tip through the bone marrow to the implant.

Inadequate bone thickness around all sides of the dental implant can cause implant failure. The thickness of the bone can be measured with a three-dimensional x-ray called a CBCT or using bone calipers to physically measure the width of the bone before placing the implant.

> ## A Discussion about Dental Implants and Bisphosphonates
>
> Most dental implant patients with a history of bisphosphonate use do well. It must be acknowledged and recognized, however, that bisphosphonates do add additional risk of failure or complications.
>
> Unfortunately, medications such as bisphosphonates taken to treat osteoporosis and osteopenia can affect implant prognosis. Under normal healthy conditions all our bone throughout our skeleton is rejuvenated by being slowly dissolved and replaced with new bone over a period of several years. In addition, the more rapid dissolving of traumatized bone and rebuilding of healthy bone is how we heal after removing teeth and placing

implants. The interruption (by bisphosphonates) of the natural removal and replacement of bone can cause trouble with tooth extractions and implant placement.

Bisphosphonate treatment prevents the loss of bone density and can help you avoid a hip fracture. Avoiding a hip fracture can prolong your life. If you are going to have dental implants placed, sometimes your doctors suggest you can take a two-month break (holiday) from taking these medications before extractions or implants to reduce your risk of implant failure and localized bone death (osteonecrosis). The decision to temporarily stop bisphosphonate use will depend on your individual risk profile. Using antibiotics and anti-microbials before procedures may also help reduce implant failure risk.

Know the facts before you decide to get implants despite bisphosphonate use:

- If you have taken bisphosphonates via an *intravenous* route, your risk of osteonecrosis, which can result in dead and dying bone after implant placement, is significant.
- If you've taken bisphosphonates *orally* for fewer than four years, your risk of osteonecrosis can be less than 1%.
- If you have taken bisphosphonates orally for less than four years but have also been taking corticosteroids, the suggestion is to work with your physician to possibly stop bisphosphonates for two months prior to implant placement and then not start bisphosphonates for another three months after.
- If you have been taking oral bisphosphonates for over four years, your physician may allow you to stop taking this drug for two months before implant surgery and for three months afterward. This may diminish your risk of osteonecrosis.

- You may wish to reduce your osteonecrosis risk by monitoring with a CTX Serum C-telopeptide blood test. All of us normally have break down and replacement of our bone cells. A CTX test measures the amount of bone turnover products in the bloodstream. Bisphosphonates affect these results.
  - If you have 150pg/ml and above on a CTX test, your risk of osteonecrosis due to bisphosphonates is low.
  - If you have between 100pg/ml to 150pg/ml, you have moderate risk of osteonecrosis due to bisphosphonates.
  - If you have less than 100pg/ml, you have high risk of osteonecrosis due to bisphosphonates.

You can do a CTX test before stopping bisphosphonates as a reference guide. Then in conjunction with your physician you can stop taking bisphosphonates and test every month. Stopping bisphosphonates can increase your CTX results around 30 points every month. Once you are above 150pg/ml then you may have less risk of osteonecrosis if you do the implant.

If you have used bisphosphonates and still are choosing to get dental implants, you may wish to do a two-stage implant procedure and leave the implant buried under the gums for longer to allow the bone to attach to the implant more securely before placing a crown on the implant.

Drugs that may reduce implant success

In addition to the bisphosphonates, the drugs listed below can negatively affect implant success. This is not an exhaustive list. Many of these drugs are available over-the-counter (without a prescription) at reduced dosages, so you may not be thinking about them as seriously as you would prescription drugs, but you should.

Gastroesophageal reflux disease is often treated with proton pump inhibitors. These can negatively affect dental implant success and include the following:

- omeprazole (Prilosec)
- esomeprazole (Nexium)
- lansoprazole (Prevacid)
- pantoprazole (Protonix)
- rabeprazole (AcipHex)
- . . . and others

Depression or anxiety is often treated with selective serotonin reuptake inhibitors which can negatively affect dental implant success and are listed here:

- citalopram (Cipramil)
- escitalopram (Cipralex)
- fluoxetine (Prozac, Oxatin)
- paroxetine (Seroxat)
- sertraline (Lustral)
- . . . and others

Rheumatoid arthritis is often treated with a combination of drugs that can affect dental implant success. Methotrexate (Rheumatrex, Trexall) is one of many.

Drugs that may help implant success

Some drugs appear to assist in the proper healing of implants. High total serum cholesterol levels increase implant and graft failures. Interestingly, statins that reduce cholesterol levels may help bone attach to the implant. Similarly, low vitamin D levels negatively impact dental implant success. So, take your vitamin D supplements.

Sinus Lift Surgery

Your sinus may not leave enough bone to place a long implant if you need to place an implant in the back of your upper arch. The choice can be to use a short implant or lift the sinus and place bone in the bottom of the sinus to allow a longer implant to be placed. This is called sinus lift surgery.

Sinus lift surgery can sometimes be done by tapping the sinus higher and adding bone through the hole that is created to place the implant. The other option is to surgically open a window in the jawbone on the side of the upper jaw. This allows your dentist to gain access to lift the sinus and fill the bottom of the space with bone. If a short implant will not be successful, your dentist must decide which one of these sinus lift surgical procedures will work best for you. Once your sinus is lifted out of the way, a longer implant can be placed. You never want to get a sinus lift done if you have an active sinus infection, a history of recurrent chronic sinus infections, a history of fungal sinus infections, uncontrolled diabetes, cystic fibrosis, a tumor in your sinus, and a few other rare conditions.

Before you get sinus lift surgery, you will want to address infections in the upper teeth and evaluate cysts in your sinus.

Since smokers have a higher failure rate with sinus lift surgery than non-smokers, you may wish to stop smoking entirely or at least fifteen days before the surgery and for six weeks after the surgery. This alleviates some of the risk associated with smoking.

After sinus lift surgery it is very common to have swelling, bruising, discomfort, minor nose bleeding, mild bleeding from the incision line, and nasal stuffiness. These problems usually resolve within a week. More serious complications include loss of graft material from the bottom of the sinus; infection; heavy bleeding; tissue dying; a connection between your sinus and your mouth developing; and occasionally even rarer issues.

Takeaways

If you have any of the issues discussed above that could affect a successful outcome and choose to get dental implants, you may wish to do a two-stage implant procedure and leave the implant buried under the gums for longer to allow the bone to attach to the implant more securely before placing a crown on the implant.

Having dental implants performed is not like having an appendix removed and then never thinking about it again. With implants you must be prepared for the likelihood of continuing complications of one type or another. Some types of implant cases have much higher rates of failure with more devastating results if they fail. Choosing an implant dentist who is not geographically close to you may cause travel and cost issues if you experience numerous unplanned follow-up appointments.

Eleven

Implant-Attached "All-on-X" Dentures

These are full-arch, permanently implant-attached dentures. Permanently implant-attached dentures are called "all-on-X" dentures, with the "X" being the number of implants chosen to support an entire arch of false teeth. The "X" is usually four, five, or six implants. "All-on-X" treatment is also occasionally called full-arch implant rehabilitation or hybrid dentures. This procedure is one of the most expensive and complex dental treatments available.

While "all-on-X" dentures are a valid choice for some patients with extremely serious problems, my opinions are presented in this chapter to make sure those considering this option understand the benefits and risks. The complete picture is not usually explained in the flashy corporate videos and advertisements or discussed in the professionally created sales presentation.

Having a full arch of artificial teeth permanently attached to four, five, or six implants is popular right now. It may be the preferred option when getting an entire arch of teeth done immediately is the objective, but it can lead to serious disappointment and disability when it fails. If you are considering getting a full arch set of artificial teeth supported by only four, five, or six implants, carefully read the facts below and make sure you are the right candidate for this therapy!

The Procedure

If you need to have most, or all, of your teeth replaced and do not want to have a removable denture or a full mouth of implants, you can choose to have a single-piece dental arch of twelve to fourteen artificial teeth made. This entire arch of teeth can be supported by only four to six long implants instead of one implant per tooth. You can have this done for both upper and lower arches at the same time or separately. This can significantly reduce the number of appointments and the unpredictability of several bone-grafting procedures. The number of implants needed is reduced because the implants used in this procedure are much longer and placed at angles in the bone to increase the amount of bone attached to each implant. The extra length helps support and distribute the chewing forces. (See Figure 11.1.)

A temporary full set of teeth is placed the same day the implants are surgically placed in the jawbone. A liquid diet is prescribed for at least three weeks because the implants cannot be traumatized and tapped on by chewing while healing. Only soft foods must be eaten for at least another month after the initial three weeks of liquid diet. Clenching and grinding on the new teeth should be avoided for many months, ideally forever.

The implants sitting in the horizontal gap between the gums and the "all-on-X" denture must be cleaned well three to four times a day with special devices and floss. The food and bacteria lodging between the gums and the "all-on-X" denture must also be scrubbed away or they will accumulate and cause bad breath.

This cleaning around the implants and of the space between the "all-on-X" denture and the gums is not easy or convenient for most people. The area that must be cleaned of food, debris, and bacteria is a large horseshoe-shaped area extending across the entire ridge of gums. An implant-retained "all-on-X" denture is not the treatment of choice for those who do not have the dexterity and serious resolve to frequently and diligently clean this area.

Additionally, the appliance and implants should be professionally cleaned at least twice a year by your dentist. These "all-on-X" dentures can only be removed by a dentist unscrewing the denture from the implants. The screws should be replaced frequently because the threads of the screws wear out and the screws will loosen and break. Replacing the screws is time consuming and costly. Most of these full-arch cases require many follow-up adjustment appointments and occasional repairs, but these implant-supported dentures can last more than fifteen years.

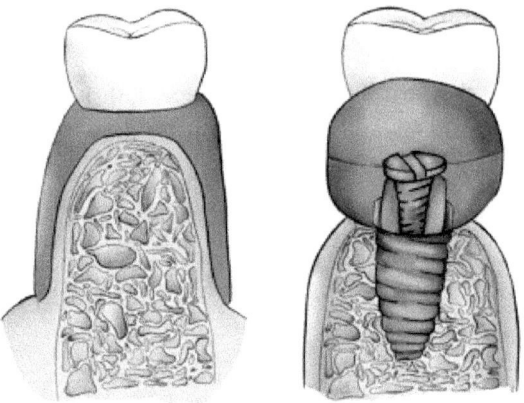

Figure 11.1 A lower denture (left) compared to a lower "all-on-X" denture on an implant.

The Advantages

The full-arch "all-on-X" option offers multiple advantages over traditional dentures as described here:

- *Chewing strength is much stronger than traditional dentures.* This can allow you to have a more nutritious diet including more difficult-to-chew vegetables and fruits. There are plenty of studies that show better diets help your longevity.

- *Implants help preserve jawbone ridge height.*

- *Implant-retained single piece dental prostheses do not slide around* over your gums when chewing or speaking.

- *No denture adhesives are needed.*

- *There is often no healing time needed for grafts to mature* before implant placement since the bone is removed to make room for the "all-on-X" denture rather than needing to be built up to support vertical implants.

- *Unlike traditional dentures, "all-on-X" dentures do not create sore spots on the gums because they are not moving and pressing on the gums with chewing efforts.*

The Risks and Disadvantages

Disastrous consequences can result when hybrid "all-on-X" dentures fail.

Individual implants have up to a 40% complication rate and sometimes do fail. Many dental appointments for repairs and maintenance must be anticipated. Permanently attaching an entire arch of twelve or more teeth to only four or five implants can pose unique risks. This large horseshoe-shaped dental appliance is attached to only a few implants compared to the number of teeth that it replaces.

Before placing the implants, space needs to be created between the upper and lower bone arches to make room for the fake gums and teeth. A significant amount of healthy bone must be removed to allow for the height of a large oval of acrylic and teeth of the "all-on-X" denture. This portion of jawbone along your entire arch must be cut away horizontally. (See Figure 11.3.) This creates a flat surface to make room for tall pink plastic gums and the artificial teeth.

There is a gap between the "all-on-X" hybrid denture and your gums to allow you to clean underneath. This gap is obvious and must be covered by your lips even when you smile your biggest smile. If your natural smile shows gum above your teeth, you will need a lot of gum height and healthy bone to be cut off.

The "all-on-X" denture has a solid oval cross section (see figure 11.2) to hold the teeth and abutment tubes that screws fit through to attach the dental prosthesis into the implants. The prosthesis must be tall and wide enough to hold the abutment tubes and not bend with biting forces.

It cannot be emphasized enough that the difficulty of daily cleaning 360 degrees around implants permanently covered up and obstructed by an "all-on-X" hybrid denture can mean leaving areas of bacteria, rotting food, and debris under the appliance. This can result in consistent bad breath.

A regular denture is U-shaped in cross section (see figure 11.2). It is easily removed to allow the food and bacteria accumulating in the concave surface to be brushed out daily.

Bone height does not need to be cut away with traditional dentures, and there is no cleaning gap that exists between the tooth crowns and the gum-colored material. A traditional denture sits on the gums and wraps down the cheek and tongue sides of the jawbone. The traditional denture gains strength from its U-shaped cross section. With a traditional denture all the jawbone is left intact and does not need to be cut down.

The diagrams below illustrate the difference between a traditional denture and an "all-on-X" hybrid denture. An obvious gap must exist between the "all-on-X" dental appliance and the patient's natural gums to allow the patient to slide cleaning devices under the appliance or food and bacteria will accumulate.

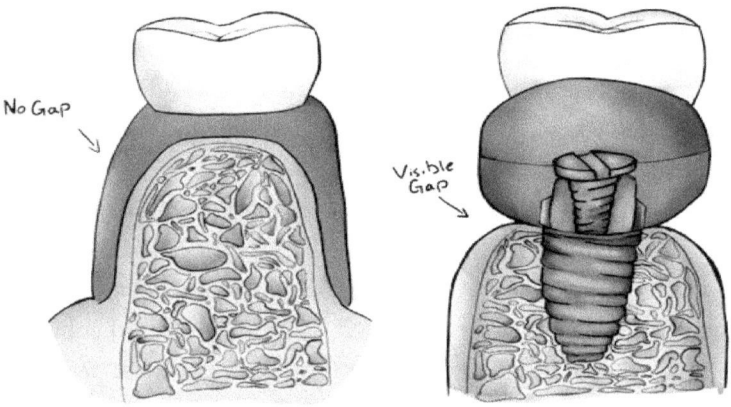

Figure 11.2. This cross section of a traditional denture on top of gum and bone (left) has no gap visible, while an "all-on-X" hybrid denture (right) has a gap.

A large amount of healthy bone must be cut away to make room for the "all-on-X" appliance. In order to not show the gap, all the bone from "A" to "B" must be cut away. (See Figure 11.3.) Because the person shown in Figure 11.4 does not have an upper lip that slides up high and shows much gum when smiling, less bone would need to be removed to hide the cleaning gap between an "all-on-X" hybrid denture and the gums compared to individuals depicted in Figure 11.6 and Figure 11.7. This gap must be hidden by your lips at rest and while smiling widely.

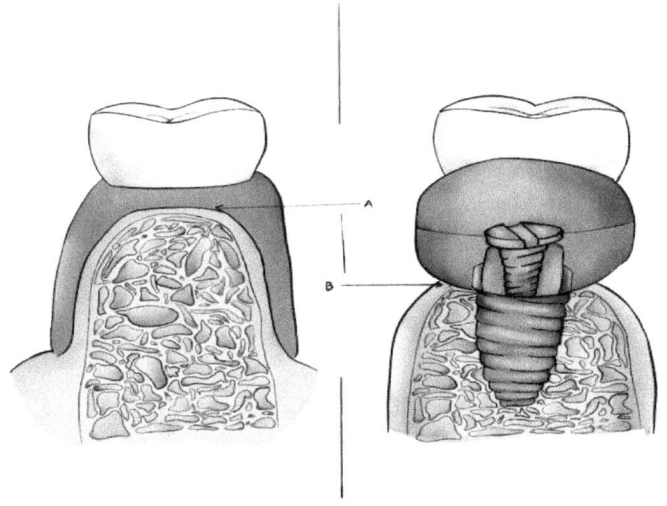

Figure 11.3. All the bone between "A" and "B" must be cut away for the "all-on-X" hybrid denture (right) to fit and hide the cleaning gap from view.

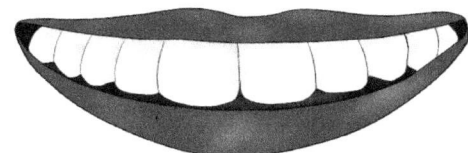

Figure 11.4. This person's smiling lip line shows no gums.

As depicted in Figure 11.5, no gap is visible with a denture; with an "all-on-X" hybrid, the lip must cover the gap.

Traditional Upper Denture   **Hybrid Denture with Upper Lip**

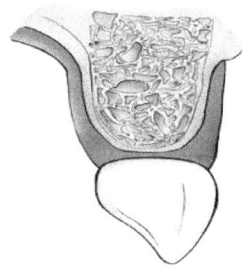
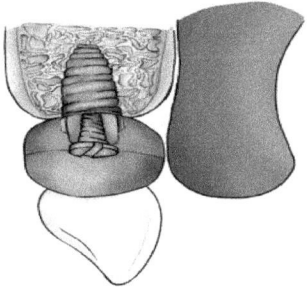

Figure 11.5. Any lip line will look normal with a denture, but lips must cover the gap created with an "all-on-X" denture.

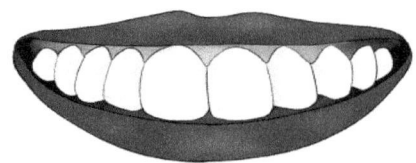

Figure 11.6. The person above shows gum while smiling, and a significant amount of bone would need to be removed to hide the cleaning gap under her upper lip to make an "all-on-X" denture.

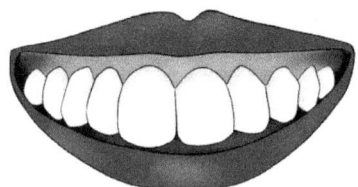

Figure 11.7. Excessive gum shows with this smile so an extreme amount of bone would need to be cut away to make an "all-on-X" hybrid denture esthetically acceptable.

The person in Figure 11.7 shows a large amount of gum above their teeth during normal activity, while smiling or talking. If this illustration looks a lot like you, you may not be a good candidate for an "all-on-X" hybrid denture because of the extra-large amount of bone that must be removed.

If the "all-on-X" hybrid denture procedure goes well, patients can be happy with this treatment choice. However, if the procedure does not go well, the results can be devastating.

Failure of an "all-on-X" hybrid denture can leave the patient with almost no jawbone ridge at all to hold new implants or a conventional denture. In addition, without the jawbone ridge, there is almost no bone left to provide a matrix to attempt to support and build more bone. These patients' ability to speak and eat can be permanently limited. Significant negative facial appearance changes also can occur immediately since the missing bone and teeth no longer support the lips and cheeks. Less bone height also makes jaw fracture more likely.

Even if the implants holding the "all-on-X" do not fail for years, you will need to deal with complications and repairs. You can be assured you will spend many more appointments visiting the dentist with an "all-on-X" denture than with a traditional denture.

Don't hesitate to ask your dentist about the risk of screws loosening; broken screws; implant failure; individual cracks forming on teeth; teeth breaking off; fracture of the entire appliance; peri-implantitis; the visible gap at the transition line between the "all-on-X" denture and your natural gums; and the challenge of cleaning well under the denture.

The highest complication rate involves problems with speech. Some studies show more than 50% of patients with "all-on-X" dentures still have speech problems years after placement.

Takeaways

Make certain that you are told and carefully evaluate the risks and benefits of your current dental options before you decide to choose an "all-on-X" denture. Many people with severely unsatisfactory dental situations will be happy initially with their "all-on-X" denture choice. "All-on-X" dentures are often retained in the mouth for many years, but these patients will need to anticipate a high prosthetic and implant complication rate requiring multiple visits to the dentist. In addition, at some point in the future, they have a good chance of facing eventual, complete arch failure, with very little remaining jawbone and few remaining esthetic and functional choices.

Twelve

Dentures

Dentures are often chosen for function and esthetics if you have lost all your teeth on one or both arches. Because dentures can replace both missing teeth and give the appearance of replacing gum height, they can be the best-looking option if you have significant bone and gum loss. If you still have some stable, healthy teeth on your upper or lower jaw, then the denture that is recommended is referred to as a "removable partial denture," as explained in the earlier chapter. Dentures make it possible for you to eat and chew when otherwise you would only have gums.

It is often said that dentures are like using a cane or a walker. You can eventually get to your destination, but the experience is not nearly as pleasant as having healthy legs and feet.

Dentures are not attached solidly to the jawbone or to teeth. They can float around in the mouth, making it difficult to eat and speak. Even if dentures seem to fit well at first, the jawbone ridge underneath the denture slowly dissolves. This is because the jawbone no longer has the active stimulation of the periodontal ligament and tooth roots pressing deep in the bone while you chew.

Dentures always become less satisfactory over time since the gum and bone ridge eventually dissolve and become so flat that the denture has nothing to hold it securely. They can be adjusted or remade when they start to have problems, but some problems cannot be fully solved. Some specific issues with dentures and some solutions are explained below.

Problems & Solutions

Denture wearers' most common complaints are that the lower denture won't stay in place and that they have pain when chewing. The following presents a discussion of these and other issues—and some possible solutions.

Chewing difficulties

Natural teeth have long roots to distribute chewing forces into the jawbone. The total surface area of all the roots is many times larger than the surface area of a denture in contact with the gums. A natural tooth can handle biting hard on food because the pressures are distributed on a long root deep in the jawbone rather than on just a small patch of gum on top of the bone.

You cannot press as hard on dentures as you could on your natural teeth. This diminished biting and chewing power makes it harder to chew food into softened, small pieces before swallowing. This often results in a denture wearer making less nutritious food choices.

It is much more difficult also for your mouth to know food position, size, and toughness when chewing with a denture. Special nerve endings exist in the ligament around tooth roots. These nerves let us know when we are unexpectedly biting into something hard. We are prevented from snapping our teeth down powerfully and breaking our teeth. These specialized nerve endings are not available on the surface where the dentures touch the gums. This lack of information from extra nerve endings makes it more difficult to chew and to know where your dentures are in your mouth.

Sore spots

Sore spots can be caused by a myriad of problems, including the surface area available to distribute chewing forces onto the jaw being much less with dentures than with natural teeth. Sore spots may also develop due to uneven bite pressures or changes in the bite; lack of saliva; inadequate cleaning of the denture; bacterial or fungal infection of surface gum tissue; poorly fitting dentures; jawbone changes that produce uneven pressure on the gums; and more.

Jawbone loss

Dentures usually get less satisfactory over time due to jawbone loss. If you choose to have dentures, you will experience significant jawbone loss over time. If the bone is not placed under pressure and tension by natural tooth roots or an implant, the height and width of your jawbone dissolves away. The bone decreases 25% in width and about 4 mm in height during the first year after teeth are extracted (if implants or bone grafts are not placed). This loss of bone diminishes your future dental choices and comfort. Bone resorption also causes additional problems because it does not occur in a perfectly smooth shape and can leave irregular, jagged areas.

This uneven bone loss means you have less support over time and need to reline or rebase your denture in about a year to assure that it will rest smoothly and firmly on the gums. Relining or rebasing will help your denture fit better, stay more stable, distribute the forces more evenly, and reduce sore spots.

The bone loss is around four times greater in the lower arch than in the upper arch during the first seven years after tooth extraction. Moreover, the bone height can resorb more than the gum tissue height leaving the gum tissue very flabby. This movable tissue wiggles and does not support the denture movement from side to side as nicely as gum tissue that tightly adheres to the jawbone.

A common solution

Dental implants with an attachment to allow the patient to snap the denture on and off improves and/or solves most of the problems described above.

Placing two, three, or four implants with an attachment to allow the patient to snap the denture on and off can help improve chewing issues and reduce problems with sore spots since the implants help support the denture. Being able to take the denture in and out to clean it daily enables you to keep your breath fresh and implants healthy. Additionally, the placement of implants allows stimulation of the bone cells in the jaw and reduces bone loss. Very few patients are unhappy with the placement of implants with removable attachments to help support their dentures.

When should these implants be placed? In order to avoid and reduce bone loss after extractions, bone grafts can be placed immediately in the sockets (spaces where the roots were) at the same time as the extraction. Implants should be placed immediately or in three or four months to help reduce bone loss. Waiting for three or four months before implant placement allows you time to carefully consider if you really need or want to get implants to support the denture.

Diminished coordination

The biting surface of denture teeth have rounded and pointy bumps (cusps) that fit into grooves on the teeth coming together from the other arch when chewing. This interdigitation helps penetrate and break down the food size. Interdigitated cusps also look more normal, make the bite more stable left to right, and reduce the amount of force the patient needs to chew effectively.

As patients with dentures grow older, their coordination and control of musculature diminishes, and they can no longer bring the upper and lower denture arches together in the same spot. The points of the cusps above do not drop into the grooves. Instead, cusp bumps hit cusp bumps and sometimes knock the denture loose and reduce effective chewing.

This problem can be addressed fairly simply: The dentist can choose flatter shaped teeth in a denture for a patient who is losing their coordination. Unfortunately, this results in less effective chewing and increases the need to go to softer and possibly less nutritious foods.

Appearance changes

Over time, due to the vertical loss of bone on the jawbone ridges, the distance between the tip of the nose and the chin becomes reduced. This bone height reduction results in a collapsed appearance and more wrinkles. Dentures need to be remade to make up for this bone loss and to retain a more youthful look.

Tissue size and shape

Bone loss does not occur uniformly, so the area of the denture that touches the gums needs to be adjusted to match the tissue changes. Denture adhesives are a temporary solution to help dentures adhere to the gum tissues. The daily removal, cleaning, and reapplication of adhesive is time-consuming and annoying. Some better solutions are described below.

Body fat changes

If you gain or lose significant weight, your tongue can add or lose fat in different proportions than your cheeks. Occasionally, a new denture needs to be made to accommodate these changes to allow the dentures to sit passively in the proper space between the cheeks and tongue.

Hydration problems

As you age, your ability to detect thirst diminishes. Older people often do not feel thirsty when they need more fluids and subsequently become dehydrated when they fail to drink. In addition, many medications that are commonly taken by middle-to-older-aged people tend to dehydrate. Dehydrated tissues make the dentures less stable and can lead to sore spots.

More than 30% of people over sixty years of age have diminished saliva due to a variety of causes. Natural saliva helps with digestion and helps protect us from bacteria. Artificial saliva products can help, although they are not as good as natural saliva. If a patient chews on a device called "Chewy Tubes," or other similar products, natural saliva is stimulated to increase in volume. You can see these "Chewy Tubes" on Amazon.

Dislodgement

If you have a denture that is knocked loose when you yawn, it is often because the extension of your lower jawbone up near your skull (coronoid process) hits the outer back edges of your upper denture. In this case you may need to see if the dentist needs to thin down the upper back and edges of the upper denture.

Unstable dentures

There are numerous potential causes for the frustrating problem of dentures not staying in place:

- You might have inadequate bone height.

- The upper denture might not be sealed across the back of your palate.

- The edges of your denture might extend too far and be lifted by muscular attachments from your cheek muscles to your jawbone.

- There might be too much loose gum tissue above your solid jawbone.

- The back teeth on one side of the arch are set too close to the back teeth on the other side of the arch leaving too little room for the tongue.

- The relationship of the upper to lower teeth may need adjustment.

- There may have been some error made when making the model of your mouth.

- If you have inadequate saliva, you will have more denture movement.

- If your jaw ridge height and shape is inadequate to stop your denture from being unstable, implants may be needed to hold your dentures.

Cheek and tongue biting

There are several situations that can cause you to bite your cheek or tongue. If the space between your nose and chin is less than it was with your original natural teeth due to tooth loss, bite collapse has occurred. Bite collapse causes your cheek to be less stretched. Since your cheek is not stretched as much as before the teeth were lost, the cheek tissue can fold in between the teeth. This can result in biting the cheek or tongue. The teeth on the denture can be placed a little taller to correct this problem.

Cheek biting can also occur if the upper teeth are not placed in the denture far enough sideways over the lower teeth to give your cheek a natural drape away from the biting activity. Another common cause can be that both of the arches of the upper and lower teeth are placed too widely toward your cheek on your denture.

If the dentures are made too narrow, tongue biting can also occur. Remaking the denture with a wider U-shape usually fixes this situation.

Swallowing problems

If you have a hard time swallowing with dentures, there are several possible reasons. The following are the most common causes: you could be dehydrated; you could have an inadequate amount of saliva due to problems with your salivary glands; the denture teeth might be placed a little too tall for your comfort; the back of your upper or lower denture might be too long; or the teeth might not be hitting evenly.

Gagging

There are many causes of gagging with dentures. Here are some: the denture is too long under your tongue; the teeth are set in the denture too tall so the teeth hit too early when you close your mouth; or the back edge of the upper denture can be too thick or can be extending too far toward the throat. Gagging can also occur if the left or right distance between lower and upper teeth is too narrow, leaving not enough room for the natural size of your tongue.

Trimming the denture and repolishing can often fix these problems. Occasionally, new dentures need to be fabricated to address these concerns.

Jaw movement

The lower jaw joint (temporal mandibular joint) and the base of the skull tend to wear and flatten as we age. This causes the lower jaw to have more left and right freedom. The lower jaw is less likely to return to the exact best spot you once used to bite your teeth together and chew. This means you need to have teeth with flatter surfaces since you cannot easily find the right spot for teeth cusps to drop into when chewing. This problem diminishes chewing efficiency and makes it hard to pulverize tough foods.

Vocal sounds

Problems with vocalizing specific sounds often occur with dentures. When you first receive dentures, these vocalization problems will be pronounced and lisps are common. Practicing the sounds that are difficult is the best way to improve your speaking with dentures. But any issues that persist after thirty days of practicing are usually due to the denture itself, and some of your sounds may not be as they were before dentures.

If your "V" sounds like an "F," the upper front teeth might be too short. Alternatively, the upper front teeth might be too long if your "F" sounds like a "V." If your "T" and "Th" sounds are not clearly distinguishable, you may need more free space between your upper and lower arches. If your "S" sounds are not clearly heard, you may have too much free space between your upper and lower arches. If you whistle when you attempt to make the "S" sound, the front teeth might be too narrow and need to be wider to expand out the space between the two canines. The opposite may be true if you hear a lisp when making the "S" sound. Other explanations for articulation inaccuracies can exist, but the above are often valuable initial changes that can help solve speech problems.

Improving the fit

If the fit is off, but you are satisfied with the way the teeth chew food and their appearance, there are three ways to change *only* the underneath side of the dentures to perfectly fit your gum ridge contours once again.

Temporary soft reline. Your dentist can add tissue-conditioning soft material to help relieve sore spots and fill in any spaces where the bone has shrunk unevenly. This will only work for a short-to-medium period of time.

A hard reline. Your dentist can also do a hard reline of your denture to compensate for bone and gum tissue that has unequally changed and resorbed under your denture. A hard reline completely replaces the inside of the denture with a new layer of acrylic.

Rebase. If a more extensive tissue-to-denture surface change needs to occur, the dentist can make an entirely new hard base that contacts the gums. This is easier and cheaper than making an entire new denture since it keeps the existing teeth.

Pneumonia

Scientific studies show patients have an increased risk of pneumonia that may be fatal if bacteria and food particles accumulate on dentures. It is in the best interest of the denture user to remove the denture and let the denture dry out at night while sleeping. Allowing the nightly drying will not cause warping with well-made dentures. Leaving the denture to dry out at night kills bacteria.

Allowing the denture to dry while you sleep reduces the volume of bacteria on the denture that can cause pneumonia when breathed into the lungs. Dentures also should be cleaned well every day with a toothbrush. If you have a hard time cleaning the denture, a dentist can reduce the nooks and crannies between the denture teeth at the gumline by covering the area with smooth clear acrylic. It is also important to clean the implants and implant-retained bar that may be supporting the dentures every day.

◈

Takeaways

Dentures are difficult to get used to and have some downsides even when they work perfectly.

Thirteen

Obstructive Sleep Apnea

In the United States at least twenty-four million people have undiagnosed obstructive sleep apnea. Obstructive sleep apnea can cause serious medical problems and daytime sleepiness. Driving while sleepy is responsible for 6,400 fatalities per year. Epidemiologic studies show people with untreated sleep apnea are more than 50% more likely to be involved in serious auto accidents—a higher rate than those who abuse alcohol.

Because it is such a serious issue, as of 2017, it is recommended that all dentists in the United States evaluate their patients for obstructive sleep apnea. Your dentist can direct you to a competent and concerned sleep physician for a diagnostic test. Only a physician can diagnose obstructive sleep apnea. Obtaining a diagnosis of obstructive sleep apnea by a physician and treatment by a physician or a dentist can improve your life and possibly prolong it.

Why & How the Problem Occurs

You can move your lower jaw in all directions because your lower jaw is not attached firmly to your skull. Your lower jaw is loosely held in place by muscles and flexible ligaments. Your tongue is attached to this movable lower jaw.

When you fall asleep, the muscles that hold the lower jaw and tongue fall into a more relaxed state. When this happens, your lower jaw falls backwards, and your tongue can either partially or fully block your throat and airway. This is particularly true if you sleep on your back. If your airway is fully or partially blocked, your body gets less oxygen to your lungs. If this reduced oxygen situation occurs often enough, your entire body can be negatively impacted by this reduced amount of oxygen. Numerous episodes of airway blockage while sleeping is called *obstructive sleep apnea.*

Low blood oxygen levels due to episodes of failing to breathe may startle a person to wake, gasp for air, and often clench their teeth together. This sudden jerking awake releases cortisol into the bloodstream and causes a jump in blood pressure and heartbeat. There is a clear association between obstructive sleep apnea and increased risk of heart attacks and stroke.

Analysis of data from an ongoing study of 1,500 participants, called the Wisconsin Sleep Cohort Study, showed untreated sleep apnea can predict problems with increased blood pressure, hypertension, stroke, depression, and mortality. (Burden of Sleep Apnea: Rationale, Design, and Major Findings of the Wisconsin Sleep Cohort Study. Sleep Med Clin, 2009; Young T., Palta M., Dempsey, J., Peppard, P., NietoF., Hla K.) Other investigators found untreated obstructive sleep apnea results in a threefold higher rate of early death by as many as five-to-seven years. (Marin JM, Carrizo SJ, Vicente E, Agusti AG. Long-term cardiovascular outcomes in men with obstructive sleep apnoea-hypopnoea with or without treatment with continuous positive airway pressure: an observational study. *Lancet.* 2005; 365:1046-53.)

The Warning Signs

There are numerous signs that may indicate you have obstructive sleep apnea:

- Sleepiness during the day
- Coughing, gasping, and choking when you wake up in the morning
- Headache first thing in the morning
- Erectile dysfunction
- Excessive trips to the bathroom during the night
- Clenching or grinding your teeth at night
- Falling asleep while watching television
- Your partner has noticed you stop breathing during sleep

- Failure to control your blood pressure with two or more medications
- Snoring
- Atrial fibrillation

Snoring is a major indicator and occurs when you have a partial airway collapse. When your airway narrows, your soft palate vibrates and creates a snoring sound. *Although snoring is suggestive of obstructive sleep apnea, not all snorers have obstructive sleep apnea.* It is best to have a physician eliminate or confirm a diagnosis of obstructive sleep apnea before getting treatment for snoring. Occasionally, too, you can have severe obstructive sleep apnea without any of these signs.

Potential Consequences

There are many potential consequences of having obstructive sleep apnea—none of them good:

- Increased risk of stroke
- Cardiovascular disease and heart attacks
- High blood pressure
- Type II diabetes
- Weight gain (stress hormones are released to tell your body to store carbohydrates)
- Memory and brain function problems
- Depression and moodiness
- Drug-resistant high blood pressure
- Numerous bodily functions and organs may perform worse due to less oxygen
- Morning headaches
- Developing earlier and worse glaucoma and possible blindness
- Erectile dysfunction

In addition to measured physiological effects like these, the disruption of sleep caused by sleep apnea, as mentioned above, can result in motor vehicle accidents due to sleepiness. (Sleep apnea was also implicated as a contributing factor in causing a serious train wreck.)

Even Las Vegas oddsmakers consider the disruption of natural sleep to result in poorer athletic performance and consider it a factor in the performance of teams that travel for sporting events. Lastly, and perhaps most irritating as a daily issue, an unhappy spouse or partner will complain about your snoring and their sleep can also be disrupted.

⌇

Diagnosing Obstructive Sleep Apnea

There are numerous types of sleep disorders. Obstructive sleep apnea is just one of those disorders. Obstructive sleep apnea is a mechanical problem with your tongue blocking your airway, while most other sleep disorders are neurological problems. A physician must interpret a sleep study called a Polysomnogram (PSG) to determine whether your sleep disorder is associated with a problem in your nervous system or only associated with your tongue blocking your airway.

Polysomnogram (PSG)

The PSG documents biophysical changes that occur during sleep to help diagnose obstructive sleep apnea and other sleep disorders. There are two main ways to get a PSG. A PSG can be obtained while you are sleeping in a sleep laboratory, away from home, where a registered polysomnographic technologist watches your activities and the test results while you are sleeping. You may also choose a home sleep apnea test which records your results while you sleep in your own bed. Both tests can allow a physician to diagnose obstructive sleep apnea. Both measure heartbeats. Both measure reductions in oxygen levels in your bloodstream via a pulse oximeter (painless device on your fingertip). But there are differences.

The laboratory sleep test provides more information and allows many more sleep-related disorder diagnoses than just obstructive sleep apnea. The laboratory sleep test, however, is much more expensive than the home sleep apnea test. This option also requires you to go to a sleep laboratory away from home and attempt to sleep with the equipment attached to you during the hours they assign. A lab PSG is mandatory if you have a sleep disorder that your physician suspects may be caused by a brain dysfunction.

The less-expensive home sleep test requires far fewer attachments to your body and is done in your own bed on your own schedule. However, because it provides less information, the home sleep test can miss some rarer, but important, disease states. Despite this, many doctors believe the home sleep test may provide a more accurate result in some ways since it represents your actual sleep behavior where you normally sleep. For these reasons, many dentists and some physicians are using the home sleep test rather than the laboratory test.

Both the laboratory sleep test and the home sleep test almost always come up with the same rating for obstructive sleep apnea. The value of the laboratory sleep test is how much more information it provides.

Your doctor will gauge results based on these and other markers:

- *Normal blood oxygen* should be at 95% concentration or higher. If you have obstructive sleep apnea or chronic lung disease like emphysema, the oxygen concentration in your blood can fall below 90% or even below 80%. When the oxygen falls below 90%, it is called hypoxemia. Hypoxemia can lead to heart problems and brain problems like dementia.

- *Apnea* is a term associated with obstructive sleep apnea. Apnea means a 90% reduction of airflow into your lungs for ten seconds or longer.

- *Hypopnea* is a 30% reduction of airflow into your lungs for ten seconds or longer with a matching 4% drop in your blood oxygen concentration level.

  Additionally, a hypopnea can be a 30% reduction of airflow into your lungs for ten seconds or longer with a matching 3% drop in your blood oxygen concentration level with an arousal or an arousal without desaturation.

- *The Apnea-Hypopnea Index (AHI)* is the combined average number of times a patient experiences apneas plus hypopneas per hour of sleep. The AHI is the standard measurement to evaluate how bad your obstructive sleep apnea is.

- *Mild obstructive sleep apnea* means you have five to fifteen events in one hour on average. An AHI score of fourteen means you can have an event as often as every four minutes. That is a lot of sleep disruption, and it is still only considered mild.

- *Moderate obstructive sleep apnea* means you have fifteen to thirty apnea plus hypopnea events in one hour on average.

- *Severe obstructive sleep apnea* means you have a total of more than thirty apnea plus hypopnea events in one hour on average. Some people have events every minute while they are trying to sleep.

Treating Sleep Apnea

Once you are diagnosed as one of the 400 million people on earth with clinically significant obstructive sleep apnea, you and your doctor need to decide how to treat it.

CPAP

The gold standard for treating obstructive sleep apnea is with a CPAP (Continuous Positive Airway Pressure) machine, which provides continuous airway pressure through an oxygen mask you wear while you sleep. There are variations of the CPAP machine including APAP, BPAP, and CPAP. For simplicity, I will just use the term CPAP. The CPAP creates incoming air pressure that pushes the tongue and throat tissues aside so that oxygenated air goes directly into your lungs. The CPAP keeps oxygen flowing to your lungs and significantly reduces the risk of a poorly oxygenated blood supply and associated health issues. CPAP also may reduce insulin resistance, which helps patients with diabetes. Some studies show over half of patients with atrial fibrillation also have obstructive sleep apnea; the success rates of treating atrial fibrillation with ablation surgery may improve if these patients are using a CPAP. If you can tolerate the CPAP, it is important to wear it all night long to get maximum benefit.

Despite CPAP being an excellent therapy, there are significant problems with CPAP use:

1. A CPAP requires electricity.

2. CPAP tubing must be cleaned to prevent infection.

3. A CPAP machine is noisy and may disturb your sleep partner.

4. While it is being used, a CPAP machine can aerosolize bacteria and viruses which can possibly infect others. This concern has been suspected as a likely contributor to the spread of Covid-19 in assisted living facilities near CPAP users.

5. Since the masks place pressure on the upper jaw, long-term use of CPAP can move the teeth position.

6. Latex allergies can develop.

7. Airflow often leaks out around the mask if not perfectly fitted to your face and can cause conjunctivitis.

8. Sinuses can dry out and cause discomfort.

9. Wearing the mask and tubing can cause you to wake up due to discomfort, causing more awake periods at night.

10. The CPAP mask should be replaced several times a year ($100 to $300 each time).

11. The CPAP machine should be replaced every three to five years ($1000 to $3000).

12. Users who need them do not use them regularly.

The biggest problem with CPAP machines is that most patients do not use them as needed. The CPAP is often knocked off or removed during the night and not replaced. The most famous CPAP study by N B Kribbs, et al. in the *American Review of Respiratory Disease* found only 46% of CPAP users studied actually wore the CPAP at least four hours on 70% of the days. *Am Rev Respir Dis. 1993 Apr;147(4):887-95.* Also, a 2016 *New England Journal of Medicine* study found that the average CPAP usage was less than 3.5 hours per night. Additionally, another article reported less than 30% of patients were using the PAP on a regular basis and over 70% were noncompliant.

This leaves the majority of CPAP patients untreated and gasping for air for over half of the night on a regular basis.

CPAP recalls

The polyester-based polyurethane materials used in many CPAP and similar Bi-level Positive Airway Pressure (BPAP) machines degrade. These toxic, potentially carcinogenic particles, foam and gas can be inhaled and swallowed. Over 10 million CPAP machines have been recalled for this problem. It has been reported that the United States Food and Drug Administration has received over 100,000 complaints and nearly 400 deaths claiming to be associated with these recalled CPAP machines and the breakdown of the foam.

An additional 17 million CPAP and BPAP machine masks were recalled in September 2022 due to the risk of magnets on the masks interfering with stents, pacemakers, and defibrillators. This can cause death or serious injury to the wearer and possibly to a caregiver with a pacemaker who is in close proximity to the mask wearer.

These serious problems physicians and patients face with CPAP therapy have dramatically increased the demand for an alternative approach to obstructive sleep apnea treatment.

Oral appliance therapy

An alternative to the CPAP is Oral Appliance Therapy (OAT) using a mandibular advancement device (MAD). There are over 100 models of oral appliances with multiple names. For simplicity, I will just use the general term mandibular advancement device. Once a physician diagnoses you with obstructive sleep apnea, a dentist can manufacture a device that fits snugly on the teeth and holds the lower jaw forward while sleeping. Since the tongue is attached to the lower jaw, the tongue is held away from the back of the throat and the airway is held open. With an open airway, you breathe more air into your lungs. Then your bloodstream and tissues will get better oxygen levels during sleep. Snoring is often reduced, and you get better sleep because there are many fewer episodes of waking up gasping for a breath. Your airway remains open, so you do not need a CPAP machine to pump air to push your tissues out of the way.

Advantages of OAT

Oral Appliance Therapy devices from your dentist do not fill your lungs with possibly cancer-causing materials, nor do they have magnets that pose other risks to patients and caregivers. Mandibular advancement devices do not produce aerosols like CPAP machines do. Mandibular advancement devices are also easily disinfected, unlike CPAP filters, tubing, and masks.

Many medical and dental providers believe also that mandibular advancement devices can be a better overall therapy for many individuals because patients use it more hours nightly. The average CPAP user wears the CPAP device about half of their sleeping hours while the average mandibular advancement device user wears their device the whole time they are sleeping.

On an hour-by-hour comparison, however, a CPAP is better than a mandibular advancement device at keeping normal oxygen levels in the blood since a CPAP machine is continuously pushing air into your lungs. Unfortunately, most patients do not use a CPAP seven hours a night or seven days a week. This may explain why some research studies have suggested, "Therapy with CPAP plus usual care, as compared to usual care alone, did not prevent cardiovascular events in patients with moderate-to-severe obstructive sleep apnea and established cardiovascular disease. (*New England Journal of Medicine* 2016; 375:919-931. Eur Respir J 2011; 37:1128-1136.) Even if the CPAP provides more perfect oxygenation while it is being worn, the benefit is significantly reduced if the average person throws it off halfway through the night. If you have a CPAP, it is important to use it all night long to get the indisputable medical benefits.

The proportion of patients continuing to use the mandibular advancement device after a year is much higher than the proportion of patients continuing to use the CPAP after a year.

You can do inexpensive home sleep tests occasionally after you start wearing the mandibular advancement device to prove you are gaining maximum oxygenation with the fewest sleep interruptions.

Mandibular advancement
devices and Covid-19

Mandibular advancement devices do not produce aerosols. Mandibular advancement devices are also easily disinfected, unlike CPAP filters, tubing, and masks. It is well established that you have a higher risk of catching Covid-19 if you are in the vicinity of a person with Covid-19 that is using a CPAP machine. Exhaled particles that remain suspended in the air can contain the Covid-19 virus. (*Nature* 2020: Aerodynamic analysis of SARS-CoV-2 in two Wuhan hospitals.) One of the initial mass deaths at a nursing home clustered around a CPAP user. This also implies other airborne diseases are possibly transmitted at greater frequency this way.

Oral Appliance Negatives

Mandibular advancement devices can move the teeth over time causing gaps between teeth, bite changes, and temporomandibular disorders. These can be minimized by using a bite aligner every day for a few minutes after removing the mandibular advancement device. There may still be some tooth movement over time despite using a bite aligner.

If a mandibular advancement device is not positioned properly, jaw discomfort can occur. A dentist experienced with mandibular advancement devices can find the best compromise between keeping your tongue far enough forward to improve your breathing during sleep and minimizing any discomfort associated with positioning the jaw forward. This calibration can take weeks and several visits. How far forward the lower jaw should be positioned with the mandibular advancement device can change over time and recalibration can be needed in the future.

There is often some initial excess salivation with wearing the mandibular device, but this nearly always disappears after a few days of wearing the device.

Oral appliance use is not effective for everyone. Around 10% of oral appliance users will not gain the desired effectiveness and do not continue to wear the device regularly.

Insurance

Do not be surprised if it is difficult to get your insurance companies to reimburse you for the all-important care of this disease. Despite a high level of non-compliance with CPAP therapy creating the need to switch to a different therapy, insurance companies will only pay for one therapy, CPAP or oral appliance, every five years. Additionally, insurance companies create obtuse and changing requirements for treatment coverage.

Dual Therapy

Sometimes it would be good for CPAP users to have a Mandibular Advancement Device as a second device. Here is why:

- CPAP users often do not bring their CPAP machine when they travel or when they know convenient electricity will not be available, such as when camping. This leaves them untreated and poorly oxygenated. A mandibular advancement device does not need electricity.

- Having a mandibular advancement device as an alternative to a CPAP could benefit members of the military. Many in the military do not have electricity next to their bunks and most people with obstructive sleep apnea snore. It could be a benefit to have a mandibular advancement device as an alternative to CPAP to reduce snoring and treat their obstructive sleep apnea when there is a limitation on electrical outlets. This is also true if users have limited time or bathroom facilities that limits their ability to clean the CPAP machine daily. Wearing a mandibular advancement device usually reduces and often eliminates snoring that could disturb the sleep of their military bunkmates. The noise from a CPAP machine might not be acceptable even when users do have electrical outlets. Having a mandibular advancement device as an alternative to a CPAP is clearly a benefit in these situations.

- Many patients can benefit by wearing both a CPAP and a mandibular advancement device simultaneously. Strong air pressure all night long is often an irritant to a CPAP user. The mandibular advancement device will hold the tongue forward keeping the airway open, which will necessitate less CPAP air pressure to be used and lead to less associated throat drying and discomfort.

Other Treatment Options

Medicine has known for decades that obstructive sleep apnea leads to a plethora of serious medical issues. This has led to many treatment approaches other than the CPAP and the oral appliance. These alternative therapies have met with varying levels of success and are discussed below.

Removing the tonsils and adenoids

Removing the tonsils and adenoids works for some children but is not shown to be nearly as effective to treat obstructive sleep apnea in adults.

Nasal surgery

Patients with sleep apnea and a deviated septum can get some improvement with a minor surgery called a septoplasty. In addition, genetically large nasal turbinate bones can block the airway in some individuals and medication to reduce inflammation around these bones or their removal can help some sleep apnea patients.

UPPP surgery

Uvulopalatopharyngoplasty surgery (UPPP) is the surgical removal of the soft palate and the uvula and adjacent throat tissues. This expands the size of the airway, reduces airway tissue blockage, and allows more air to easily flow to the lungs. More oxygen means healthier tissues and a more rejuvenating sleep, reducing grogginess. This surgery has been shown to improve cardiovascular outcomes and reduce motor vehicle accident risk. This surgery is very painful for the patient and has a poor long-term success rate. The short-term results were reported in one study as "… 30% of our patients were markedly improved, 33% somewhat improved, and 37% unimproved." (*Wetmore, SJ., Laryngoscope. 1986 Jul;96(7):738-41.*) In unique situations, however, this is a good therapy.

Tongue surgery

Tongue surgery is a more extreme option that involves numerous sequential surgical appointments to remove sections of the back of the tongue. This takes two to five surgeries over six to nine months. These procedures can help reduce the problem with obstructive sleep apnea, but they can result in difficulty with speech and other speaking issues. Since many taste buds are in the tongue, surgically removing part of the tongue results in a diminished sense of taste. Problems with swallowing and gagging can also occur after tongue surgery.

Hypoglossal nerve stimulator

A hypoglossal nerve stimulator is a pacemaker-type device that is surgically placed in your chest with a wire that detects chest muscle breathing effort and a wire that extends up your neck to stimulate the tongue nerve. Stimulating the tongue nerve (hypoglossal nerve) contracts the tongue and pulls the tongue forward off the back of the throat. This opens the airway to help you breathe while you sleep. You turn the device off with a remote control when you wake up. Plenty of patients that have this treatment get significant improvement in their obstructive sleep apnea. Negative aspects can include infection, tongue abrasion, discomfort, need for a second repositioning surgery, need for surgical removal or replacement, need for battery replacement, trouble getting an MRI, nerve injury, dry mouth, facial incision scarring, and more rarely tongue paralysis and speech issues. Despite this list of negatives, this device is the best choice to treat obstructive sleep apnea for plenty of people, especially if it prevents a stroke, heart attack, or early death. When you breathe while sleeping your tongue gets a small electrical shock and the stimulated muscles pull your tongue forward. This procedure works because it pulls the tongue off the back of the throat when you are sleeping. This opens the airway so the air you breathe through your nose can flow unimpeded down into your lungs.

The placement of a hypoglossal nerve stimulator involves an extensive surgery. Your body heals tightly to the wires from your chest to your tongue. This is fine unless you need to remove it at a later date. Removing these wires involves cutting out the wires and can cause damage to your nerves and throat tissues.

Additional surgeries are needed to replace the batteries each time they wear out.

The presence of the hypoglossal nerve stimulator can make a good MRI impossible or more difficult to achieve if you need an MRI of your head and neck area in the future. Make sure your doctor chooses a device that does not interfere with MRIs. Of course, if the hypoglossal nerve stimulator is your best choice to treat your obstructive sleep apnea, the risks of the surgery can be worth it to avoid all the cardiovascular problems associated with not breathing or sleeping well.

Tongue-retaining device

If you have no teeth, or just a few teeth, a mandibular advancement device usually will not work. You can use a *tongue-retaining device* which is a suction cup type device attached onto the tip of your tongue to hold your tongue forward. It is worn like a pacifier at night. This tongue-retaining device is also called a tongue-stabilizing device and can hold your tongue off the back of your throat. This device became well-known when it was used to help snorers from bothering adjacent sleepers in temporary group housing after the Japanese earthquake and Fukushima Daiichi nuclear power plant incident in 2011. The tongue-stabilizing device causes lip soreness, tongue soreness, and disturbed sleep due to irritation, but can provide a reasonably good benefit if you are among the fewer than 10% that can continue to use it. This device cannot be adjusted, but it is an inexpensive option to try if you do not have enough teeth to hold a mandibular advancement device.

Tracheotomy

Tracheotomy was first shown to reduce the complications and symptoms of obstructive sleep apnea in 1970 and 1973. Symptoms like daytime drowsiness "disappeared." Surgically opening a hole in your trachea works because it opens your airway below where your tongue is blocking the flow of air. Luckily, we currently have better therapy.

Palatal Expansion

If you create more room for the tongue by expanding the palate, the tongue has less pressure to fall backwards while you sleep. This irreversible therapy can improve sleep apnea.

Muscular Therapy

There are many muscular exercises that can provide minor improvements. The one exercise that has been shown to be more than marginally beneficial is to take up playing a wind instrument.

Positional therapy

Wearing a positional therapy device on your back that keeps you sleeping on your side can help with snoring and obstructive sleep apnea. A sleep test will tell you which side is best for you to sleep on. Tangentially, if you have GERD or acid reflux, the acid coming up into your throat causes heartburn and can wake you up. If you have this problem, you may wish to sleep on an elevated bed or on your left side because stomach acids have a harder time flowing out of the stomach and towards your throat because of the angle of the esophagus coming out of the stomach.

Takeaways

Obstructive sleep apnea can damage your health and shorten your life. A CPAP machine is the most efficient way to deliver oxygen to your lungs. Unfortunately, people are often intolerant of the CPAP machine. Those who need it do not wear it often enough or long enough to maximize its potential. If you have *severe* obstructive sleep apnea, you should get a CPAP machine and try to use it all night, seven days a week.

If you have *mild-to-moderate* obstructive sleep apnea, you may wish to try a mandibular advancement device first to improve your sleep and oxygenation of your body.

A mandibular advancement device is fairly comfortable, and patients usually wear it all night long and seven days a week. The overall difference in usage might make a mandibular advancement device the most effective way to treat obstructive sleep apnea in most patients. This is especially true in mild-to-moderate cases of obstructive sleep apnea.

Both CPAP and oral appliance therapies are non-invasive therapies that can be tried before moving on to surgical options. There are lots of treatment choices because there is no perfect treatment for obstructive sleep apnea.

Fourteen

Prevention

The average person touches their teeth together thousands of times every day. The maintenance and care of anything you use thousands of times a day cannot be delegated to a dentist who only sees you once or twice a year. It is important you do your own daily maintenance, or you are likely to be at risk for tooth loss.

Avoiding Periodontal Disease

As we discussed in chapter one, most adult teeth are lost due to periodontal disease. Our teeth are always naturally coated with bacteria. If the bacteria are not removed, they build a sticky attachment to the tooth that helps the bacteria stay in position. Bacteria die after a few days and when this happens salts and minerals from saliva deposit in their cell walls and harden into calculus that firmly attaches to the tooth. This calculus is porous and forms a home for more bacteria. It is difficult to remove with just brushing and flossing.

The hardening of bacterial bodies into hard calculus takes at least forty-eight hours. This means if you go longer than forty-eight hours between a good brushing and flossing, calculus will start forming. Try to brush and floss every day, but especially never miss two days in a row. Even brushing every day, no one can brush and floss perfectly every time, especially considering that some areas are difficult to reach and bacteria will also build up under our gums.

Deep periodontal pockets must be cleaned each visit

Because it is difficult to perfectly clean all areas of your teeth by brushing and flossing at home, you will miss some hard-to-reach areas. The bacteria you miss will grow under the gumline into the spaces next to the teeth and can eventually cause periodontal pockets. These areas will build up bacterial colonies and calculus that must be cleaned out and scraped off the teeth professionally by a dentist or hygienist.

These pockets are measured by dentists and hygienists as a record of the health of your mouth. Most people with periodontal pockets shallower than 5 millimeters (mm) do well with good home care and professional dental hygiene cleanings every six months. Going longer than six months between these cleanings will significantly add to the risk of advancing gum disease, bone loss, and forming pockets deeper than 5 mm.

If you have a pocket greater than 5 mm, your risk of periodontal disease and resultant tooth loss will increase alarmingly. Your regular interval of cleanings usually must change from six months to every three months (occasionally sooner) once you get pockets greater than 5 mm. This is because the deeper spaces still exist after a perfect professional cleaning; bacteria will recolonize those spaces over time. Your daily brushing and flossing efforts cannot reach that far under the gums. You can slow down the bacterial growth by doing excellent home care, but eventually bacteria will get there.

Once a periodontal pocket is cleaned out by a meticulous hygienist, it takes around ninety days for destructive bacteria to take hold. During those ninety days, normal bacteria slide under the gums and grow into an initial colony of oxygen-loving bacteria. Once those bacteria consume most of the oxygen, the colony gets replaced by a mostly oxygen-hating destructive bacterial species. At around ninety days, the colony will have grown large enough to start the destruction of gum tissue and bone. This destruction of bone is called periodontitis and is the main reason why adults lose their teeth.

Takeaway

Once you get periodontal pockets deeper than 5 mm, you may need a professional cleaning at around every ninety days to control further bone loss. Just polishing the teeth will not stop the disease from progressing.

Root planing and/or periodontal surgery

The most destructive bacterial species hate oxygen and hide in deep unoxygenated areas in your mouth. The bacteria are particularly prevalent when the space gets to be 5 millimeters (mm) or deeper. Unfortunately, 5 mm is the deepest space that excellent dental hygienists and periodontists can perfectly clean.

Should regular cleanings fail to reduce your periodontal pockets to 5 mm or less, you may opt for root planing and/or periodontal surgery to prevent eventual tooth loss. During root planing, the dentist or dental hygienist uses specially shaped instruments to remove bacteria, biofilm, and calculus from under the gums. Reducing these pockets to a cleansable 5 mm or less is the main objective.

If these deep pockets remain inflamed and impossible to clean even with frequent office visits with your hygienist and/or root planing by your dentist, periodontal surgery may need to be performed. Periodontal surgery allows visualization and removal of calculus and bacteria in deep areas. Periodontal surgery can result in a reduction in pocket depth to a shallower, easier-to-clean periodontal pocket and an eventual return to dental health.

Prevention of Cavities in Adults

Bacteria that sit in grooves on your teeth eat sugars from your food and produce acid. This acid will dissolve the surface of your teeth, creating cavities (dental caries).

Food and drink

What we drink and eat can affect our dental health. Follow these simple guidelines to help prevent cavities:

- Avoid sugary and sticky foods that stick to your teeth and feed the bacteria in your mouth.
- Limit sugary drinks. Even 100% fruit juices and energy drinks have a lot of sugar.
- If you eat or drink sugary foods, consume them with your main meals.
- Reduce the frequency of meals and snacks. The bacteria produce acid rapidly after each meal or snack. If you eat fewer times a day, your

incidence of cavities will decrease. Said another way, slowly drinking one soda all day long is much worse for your teeth than drinking three sodas in an hour would be.

- Limit breath mints between meals. They are usually full of sugar and feed the bacteria creating cavities. You can also look for sugar-free mints or candy instead.

- Drink water after meals to dilute the sugars and remove bits of food.

Saliva helps wash away bacteria and contains protective components that help fight bacteria that cause cavities. If you do not drink enough fluid, you will not produce adequate saliva. You should drink six to eleven cups of fluid a day. This amount must be adjusted upward for hotter and dryer environments, larger people, and increased exercise levels. Also, men need more water than women.

Research has revealed that we tend to be less aware of thirst as we age, and subsequently drink less water than ideal. This causes us to have less saliva. Hundreds of different medications also reduce our saliva and cause us to have drier mouths. Fight against this by ensuring your water intake is enough. Saliva substitutes can be recommended, but their value is limited. Older adults, especially those in nursing homes, get root cavities due to not drinking enough water and limited access to good oral care. A single topical application of silver diamine fluoride stops over 80% of these cavities from getting worse. It is amazing and inexpensive.

Eating food creates an acidic environment in your mouth. The extra acid puts your teeth in a momentarily softer and weakened state. Wait an hour after eating or drinking acidic beverages like coffee before brushing and flossing: this allows your saliva to return your mouth to an alkaline state. This will reduce extra wear on your teeth.

Tap water with fluoride and fluoridated toothpaste also help reduce cavities.

Brush and floss

Brush and floss well at least twice daily and especially before bedtime. Oral-B oscillating, round-headed electric toothbrushes or sonic electric toothbrushes by Phillips and other companies work about 20% better at removing bacteria than a manual toothbrush. These brushes also have timers that motivate you to brush the proper length of time. However, do not use a scrubbing motion with these electric toothbrushes because this will make your brushing ineffective and can damage your teeth and gums. With electric toothbrushes, you must brush one tooth at a time instead of using a scrubbing motion. Follow the instructions that come with the brush or what your dentist or hygienist tells you. You should avoid cheap vibrating toothbrushes that shake the whole toothbrush rather than only the bristles. These toothbrushes make you think they are working, but the bristles do not end up where they need to be.

The key to picking a good electric toothbrush is finding a name brand like the ones mentioned above. Choose the brushes with separate brush heads that include the word "oscillating" in the product description. Additionally, I believe the heads with bristles in a round circle are more effective than the ones in a rectangular shape. Spending more money here will help you avoid serious troubles later. The term "oscillating" is the easy way to determine what to buy.

Your toothbrush or electric toothbrush head must be replaced around every three months. Most people only replace them slightly more often than once a year and that results in poor cleaning efforts when you brush your teeth. Make sure to purchase high-quality brushes that say "soft" on them, because cheap brushes can have sharp, stiffer bristles that can damage your gums.

Even though electric toothbrushes may be more efficient at plaque removal, sometimes they can pose problems with usage by senior adults. Some adults of advanced age cannot identify where the on/off button is by sight or touch, or do not have the dexterity to manipulate the button. This must be evaluated when helping them choose the best oral hygiene device for them. Topical silver diamine fluoride can control sensitivity and stop cavities if these senior adults with oral hygiene issues start to develop root cavities.

Use fluoridated toothpaste. Make sure to use a toothpaste with the American Dental Association seal of acceptance to make sure the product has been tested independently and does not contain sugar. Fluoride can help prevent dental cavities and even slow the progress of tiny cavities that have already started. See a dentist frequently. Professionally applied fluoride treatments can help reduce cavities in children and adults. Occasionally a stronger prescription fluoride toothpaste for daily use may be indicated. Fluoridating water supplies for entire populations is currently under debate.

The most important things to remember when picking toothbrushes is to pick name brands that have the ADA (American Dental Association) seal on them and choose brushes that have soft or extra-soft bristles to avoid scratching your gums and wearing away any exposed roots. Additionally, see your dentist at least every year and more often if you have a history of cavities or gum disease.

Orthodontics

Straightening out crooked and crowded teeth and poor jaw relations help you keep your teeth. Nicely aligned teeth make cleaning efforts easier to perform by you, your dentist, and dental hygienist. Teeth in an ideal natural curve also make it easier to detect cavities and gum disease while the problems are small.

If you are going to have orthodontics as an adult, however, make sure to get a good examination for gum disease *before* braces are initiated. Orthodontics will magnify bone loss if you have untreated gum disease. I have had adult patients referred to me to attempt to save their newly straightened teeth they are likely to lose due to excessive periodontal bone loss during orthodontics. Discovering if you have gum disease and treating it before orthodontics can minimize risk of bone and tooth loss during orthodontics. Seeing an excellent dental hygienist more often than every six months during orthodontic treatment can help prevent periodontitis worsening during orthodontics.

If the way your teeth come together is uneven, you can get a muscular spasm in your jaw joint area or temporalis muscle.

Having orthodontics to correct a crooked smile is valuable for numerous health and social reasons. However, there are several things you should be aware of that can arise during orthodontics. The likelihood of having negative issues increases with the length of treatment time and can be minimized by making sure you stay on your prescribed schedule of visits to the orthodontist. In addition, you will want to keep your teeth as clean as possible and see your general dentist at least twice a year.

Concerns to be aware of during orthodontics.

- It is natural to have some discomfort when the orthodontic appliances are inserted and adjusted. Taking non-prescription pain medication almost always controls this.

- Wearing a removable or non-removable retainer after orthodontics has been completed is usually mandatory to prevent relapse.

- Cavities or tooth decalcification around the orthodontic appliances can occur if these areas are not kept exceptionally clean.

- Periodontal disease can occur if you don't see the dentist to clean the teeth while wearing braces.

- Occasionally, the tips of tooth roots can resorb during orthodontics.

- Jaw joint problems can occur during orthodontics.

- Some minor adjustments to the bite may be necessary at the end of orthodontics.

- Other problems can occur during orthodontics, but they are rare.

Dental Problems in Children

Follow these simple guidelines to prevent dental problems in children.

- Make sure there is the correct concentration of fluoride in your drinking water. Hot climates need a smaller concentration because people drink more water.

- Have children take fluoride supplements if your community does not fluoridate the water supply.

- Have sealants or fluoride varnish placed on the biting surfaces of the teeth with deep grooves. Topical placement of silver diamine fluoride may work even better.

- Where teeth have been removed, space maintainer devices are needed to minimize both the tilting of adjacent teeth into that space and the need for orthodontics. The space maintainer will also help to keep the palate area and jaws as large as possible to maintain the natural space for the tongue. Keeping a natural, ideal amount of space for the tongue reduces the risk of developing obstructive sleep apnea. If the dental arch space is reduced, the tongue is pressed backwards into the throat, limiting the size of the airway.

- Have an orthodontist check your child's bite by age six.

- Do fillings and crowns on baby teeth with cavities rather than extract them if possible. The reason is to help the palate and jaws stay as large as possible to reduce the risk of developing bite problems and obstructive sleep apnea. Early diagnosis of cavities can prevent a lifetime of dental problems including bite defects, obstructive sleep apnea, temporomandibular disorders, and appearance issues.

Takeaway

See a dentist often enough to catch cavities when the cavities are small and avoid the domino effect leading to more and more dental treatment. Use fluoride toothpaste and have sealants placed or silver diamine fluoride applied if indicated.

Protecting Your Teeth Against Injury

After gum disease and cavities, the third most likely way to lose teeth is due to the types of trauma described below:

- Falls and automobile accidents are a significant cause of tooth loss.

- A surprising number of teeth are lost chewing on hard substances such as ice, nut shells, or using teeth to bite or tear open lids or plastic bags. These activities can lead to tiny cracks that can trap food stains and be unesthetic. Tiny cracks can also eventually lead to tooth fracture. It is best to avoid this behavior.

- Many people break their front teeth drinking beer from a glass bottle when they get bumped in a crowded bar.

- Heat and chemical trauma from vaping and hookah use can damage your oral tissues and occasionally lead to oral cancer.

- Lip rings or tongue studs destroy the adjacent gum tissue and can rapidly lead to tooth loss.

The following are two safeguards that can help prevent serious injury: mouthguards and night guards.

Mouthguards

Teeth can be lost due to a physical injury while playing sports. It is important to wear *mouthguards* when partaking in contact sports.

Night Guards

When you are asleep, your sensitivity to how much pressure is placed on your teeth diminishes. Clenching or grinding your teeth is called bruxism. If you are asleep, you do not get the same warning that you are biting too hard as if you were awake. Many dentists recommend wearing a *night guard* to cover the teeth and prevent fragile crowns or veneers from breaking during heavy clenching or grinding.

But before using a night guard because you grind your teeth, you will want to rule out sleep apnea. Some studies show that 70% of bruxism is caused by sleep apnea. If you have obstructive sleep apnea, the extra volume of acrylic from the night guard in your mouth leaves less room for your tongue. This can add to the tendency of your tongue to fall backward while sleeping, blocking your airway, which makes it more difficult to breathe and magnifies obstructive sleep apnea. Make sure you get tested for sleep apnea before wearing a night guard. Quite often a mandibular advancement device can be a better choice than a traditional night guard.

Don't Ignore a Swelling or Lump

If you get a swelling on your face that extends down your neck or toward your eye, you must see a dentist or your physician immediately because the swellings can be life-threatening.

If you notice any lumps or ulcers in your mouth that do not go away in two weeks, you should see a dentist to help determine if it is oral cancer. The incidence rates of oral cancer have been increasing since 2007.

Fifteen

Local Anesthesia & Laughing Gas

You can help avoid painful situations by understanding how local anesthesia and laughing gas work and the situations where they fail to work.

Local anesthetics are drugs that are deposited near the nerves of concern. The ideal effect is pain-free dentistry. There are several types of local anesthesia and different situations call for different local anesthetics. (Generic local anesthetics listed below are lower case and brand names are upper case.)

Currently, the main drugs used for local anesthesia and dentistry are articaine HCl (Septocaine), bupivacaine HCl (Marcaine), lidocaine HCl (Xylocaine, Octocaine), mepivacaine HCl (Carbocaine, Isocaine), and prilocaine HCl (Citanest).

In the past, Novocaine was widely used. Today the drug is no longer used because many people were allergic to it, and it does not work as fast or last as long as the current drugs.

Different local anesthetics create their numbing effect for varying amounts of time. Mepivacaine has a short duration of fifteen to forty-five minutes. Bupivacaine can last two to over four hours on occasion. Most of the time pain-numbing drugs we currently use for local anesthesia work well and allow for pain-free dentistry.

Challenges and Risks of Local Anesthesia

Local anesthetics are usually effective in making dentistry fairly comfortable, but there are significant situations where local anesthesia is woefully inadequate and can be troublesome.

Infection

Almost all teeth are easy to get numb, except when you have a severe infection in a tooth. If you have a bad infection, the area of the infection becomes more acidic. When areas are acidic, there is a high concentration of hydrogen ions, which causes local anesthetics to be less effective. The extra hydrogen ions prevent the local anesthetic from soaking into the nerve to block pain messages. Specifically, too many hydrogen ions cause most of the anesthetic to shift mostly into a chemical state (cationic form) that cannot diffuse into the nerve and block pain impulses. Unfortunately, this means when there is a severe infection and we need the local anesthetic to work exquisitely, it often works imperfectly. Don't wait until you are in pain with a bad infection to see the dentist.

Mandibular (lower) molars

Sometimes the lower molars are difficult to numb. This is because the path of the nerve that supplies the lower molars is further from the surface, so it is easier to miss. Also, the location of the nerve varies in position from person to person. Even if lower molars do not get numb on the first try, usually these teeth can be numbed by depositing the local anesthetic drug in a slightly different place or using a different injection approach.

Chewing on numb tissues

An occasional negative aspect of local anesthesia is that the numbing of tissues inside the mouth may cause a patient to accidentally chew on their tongue or cheek. If you are getting local anesthesia for the first time, your dentist needs to warn you not to chew on the "funny-feeling" tissues in your mouth after you receive an anesthetic. If this is a risk for someone you are caring for, ask their dentist to consider using a local anesthetic reversal agent at the end of the procedure to minimize the length of time the tissues are numb and feel odd.

Heart palpitations

Heart palpitations after dental injections occur because the local anesthetic usually includes adrenaline (epinephrine). The epinephrine in the anesthetic speeds up your heartbeat momentarily and is why many people feel they have a reaction to local anesthetics.

Almost all local anesthetics dilate blood vessels. The dilated vessels bring extra blood flow in the area. This causes the local anesthetic to be washed away quickly, which leads to a short duration of effectiveness. To make local anesthetics last longer and to avoid needing reinjection, blood vessel constrictor medications (vasoconstrictors) are included in the anesthetic. Having a vasoconstrictor in the local anesthetic not only makes the duration of the anesthetic longer, it also creates a better numbing effect. The most common blood vessel constrictor used is epinephrine (adrenaline). Another vasoconstrictor is levonordefrin (Neo-Cobefrin). Some local anesthetics work better with one vasoconstrictor rather than another.

Fortunately, if after an injection the uncomfortable feeling of palpitations and sweating occurs, it almost always goes away within ninety seconds.

Nerve damage

Physical damage by the anesthetic needle cutting into the nerves can occur but is rare. The most common nerve damage is to the inferior alveolar nerve, which goes to the lower lip, tongue, gum, and teeth. Statistics show inferior alveolar injections cause nerve damage one out of 26,762 injections. (Pogrel MA, Thamby S. J Am Dent Assoc. 2000;131(7):901-7.)

Allergic reactions

True allergic reactions to current local anesthetics are exceedingly rare, but possible. Local anesthetics used in dentistry are incredibly safe. Adverse drug reactions happen way less than 1% of the time. Although reports of allergic reactions are not uncommon, they often result from a patient's nervousness about the injection or feeling the effects of adrenaline included in the anesthetic. The occurrence of real, reproducible, allergic reactions to commonly used dental local anesthetics is almost nonexistent.

Overdosage

The main risk of having local anesthetic is if you are given too much at once. Maximum recommended dosages of anesthetics are rarely approached except in large dental cases when your dentist does all four areas of your mouth at once. These big procedures can require multiple injections and care must be taken to avoid using too much local anesthetic. Smaller people and children are at higher risk.

Laughing gas

Nitrous oxide (N_2O) is a colorless gas that provides anxiety reduction. It is also called "laughing gas." You will still need a local anesthetic to do dental procedures, since nitrous oxide does not provide much pain relief.

The amount of laughing gas you breathe in is adjusted to your personal responsiveness and sensitivity to the gas. You start with 100% oxygen and the nitrous oxide is added in small increments until you are comfortable and relaxed. It is very safe because in addition to the nitrous oxide, you are always breathing in a much higher-than-normal concentration of oxygen than is found in room air. The nitrous oxide machine will sound an alarm if the tank runs out of oxygen.

The effect of nitrous oxide starts within twenty seconds, and it takes two to three minutes to take full effect. This process may start with lightheadedness, tingling in your hands and a warm feeling. You will become relaxed and can also experience euphoria.

Negative aspects of laughing gas

Nitrous oxide does not stay in your blood. This is usually a good thing, but this means when you turn off the laughing gas at the end of your treatment, the gasses in your lungs, including nitrous oxide and carbon dioxide, are exhaled immediately. Carbon dioxide is the stimulus that tells us to breathe. This sudden exhaling of carbon dioxide can cause you to forget to take breaths for a few moments, which can give you a headache. To avoid this, you are told to take a few big breaths, and 100% oxygen is given to you for a few extra minutes after the nitrous oxide stops flowing.

Uncomfortable symptoms can occur. If the concentration of the nitrous oxide is adjusted beyond ideal for you, sweating, nausea, dizziness, loss of balance, leg weakness, impaired thought processes, poor memory of events, disorientation, dissociation, and possibly vomiting can occur. Dropping back the concentration of the laughing gas rapidly reduces these negative aspects. Different people need different concentrations of nitrous oxide—it is the dentist's job to watch your breathing and adjust accordingly. Also, it is always good to avoid a large meal before using laughing gas to minimize any vomiting.

The effects of nitrous oxide last only for about five minutes after you take the mask off. Studies indicate it is safe to drive a car after fifteen minutes.

If you are pregnant, you should be concerned that some studies suggest that nitrous oxide could present risks to the developing unborn baby. If you are pregnant, it may be prudent to stay clear of nitrous oxide. (These same risks can be passed along to any pregnant dental staff member who may be breathing the exhaled nitrous oxide that escapes into the treatment room.)

If you cannot breathe through your nose, nitrous oxide is not for you.

If you have chronic obstructive pulmonary disease or emphysema, you should avoid laughing gas. These conditions change your natural stimulus to breathe, and nitrous oxide use may compromise your normal feeling that you need to take a breath.

If you are taking psychotherapeutic drugs, you may wish to avoid the interactions with nitrous oxide. These drugs can include lithium, tricyclic antidepressants, and others. Double check with your physician and dentist about safety with nitrous oxide.

Do not abuse nitrous oxide. Heavy, repeated recreational use of nitrous oxide can cause irreversible physical problems and resultant permanent nerve damage due to nitrous oxide interfering with the metabolism of Vitamin B12. These problems can include being unable to walk, bowel and bladder incontinence, and falling down.

Sixteen

Pain Control

Local anesthesia and laughing gas are wonderful for eliminating discomfort during a dental procedure, but we often need pain control before and after the dental visit.

The Varieties of Pain

There are many different types of dental pain. It is valuable to describe any pain you have accurately by type and intensity to obtain the best diagnosis and care.

Sensitivity

Sensitivity is the type of pain that can be intense and occurs suddenly when your teeth are exposed to cold or hot foods and liquids, or even cold air. This is usually caused by a cavity or exposed roots.

Biting pain

Biting pain occurs when you chew on something, and a sharp jolt of pain occurs. It is valuable to notice if your pain occurs when biting down or upon releasing after you bite. If the pain happens when you release your bite, it often indicates you have a crack. When you bite down with a cracked tooth, the pieces separate. When you open again, the tooth pieces come back together and it hurts because the tooth's nerve gets pinched. Biting pain can also indicate a cavity or a restoration that is too high for your bite.

Throbbing pain

Throbbing pain is usually continuous but may be relieved temporarily with cold or hot water. This is usually serious and should be diagnosed and treated as soon as possible. Throbbing pain is occasionally an easy-to-diagnose problem. Sometimes the pain can seem to originate from a specific tooth but is actually from a tooth above or below on the same side, but rarely is left-side pain originating from the right side and vice versa.

Generalized pain

Generalized pain can originate from the trauma of a surgery, from jaw joint problems, or from a neurological source. Another simple example of generalized pain is when you injure yourself, such as when getting hit in the head, and an entire side of your jaw hurts.

Medications for Pain

Over-the-counter pain control after your procedure is usually more effective than prescription drugs. Numerous research papers show alternating acetaminophen (Tylenol) with ibuprofen (Advil, Motrin) provides better pain relief than most highly addictive prescription pain killers.

Additionally, a recent study showed non-prescription naproxen sodium (Aleve) 440 mg was better at reducing pain and provided longer relief than prescription hydrocodone plus acetaminophen 10/650 mg after impacted wisdom tooth removal.

While these over-the-counter medications might be the best choices for pain control, no medication is perfectly safe. Depending on the dose and length of usage, ibuprofen can negatively affect the stomach, kidney, and heart. Tylenol is particularly tough on the liver in high doses.

Avoid *unprescribed* blood-thinning medications before surgery. Do not take ibuprofen or other nonsteroidal anti-inflammatory drugs (NSAIDs) or aspirin before dental appointments as they can cause increased bleeding during and after any dental surgery. It is better to take acetaminophen (Tylenol) to reduce anticipated discomfort.

Keep taking *prescribed* blood thinners unless you are cleared by your physician to stop them temporarily. Your physician may have prescribed a daily aspirin regimen or other blood thinners to help reduce your risk of a first or second heart attack or stroke. Stopping these therapies abruptly can cause a rebound effect significantly increasing blood clot formation and possible heart attack or stroke.

If you take ibuprofen or other nonsteroidal anti-inflammatory drugs (NSAIDs) while on daily aspirin, your normal increased risk of bleeding increases even more. Make sure to discuss these medications and possible temporary alternatives with your dentist or physician before planned oral surgery.

Seventeen

Non-Dental Causes
of Tooth Pain

This happens far too often: a patient will have multiple root canals or extractions performed, separated by weeks at a time, in an attempt to alleviate pain that is never eliminated. This nightmarish situation is because the patient had a non-dental cause of tooth pain that went undiscovered. This scenario could possibly have been avoided with a little extra knowledge of the potential non-dental causes of tooth pain not necessarily found in a dental health history form. You might want to make sure you understand the issues described here and tell the dentist if you have one of these conditions and have pain that is hard to diagnose.

Your Tooth Pain May Originate Elsewhere

Tooth pain usually originates from tooth and gum issues, but if the examination of the teeth and gums does not lead to an obvious diagnosis, you must consider other causes to eliminate unnecessary dental treatment.

Over five million people a year in the United States have tooth pain *not* originating from problems with the teeth. Some of the things you and your dentist must consider are described below.

Temporomandibular disorders (TMD)

If the way your teeth come together is uneven or you grind your teeth, you can get a *muscular spasm in your jaw joint area* or temporalis muscle. This spasm can cause pain that appears to be from a tooth and can mislead you to believe the tooth is the cause of your pain. See a TMD specialist.

Heavy localized biting forces

Heavy localized biting forces can cause tooth pain. If a tooth is higher than ideal or your body likes to bite on one area preferentially, the trauma to the tooth/teeth in that area can cause pain. Your dentist can evaluate the heaviness of your bite on a painful tooth and reduce the height of the tooth a little bit. This most frequently happens after a new crown is placed. If you have tooth or jaw pain after a new crown, let your dentist know and they should be able to adjust or remake the crown.

Infection in the sinuses

An infection or inflammation in your sinuses can mimic tooth pain. The nerves of the upper teeth can travel into your sinuses and be irritated by sinus infections. This can occasionally be diagnosed by your dentist putting a topical anesthetic on a Q-tip® and gently sliding it up your nose. The anesthetic soaks into your sinuses and you can see if the pain disappears. You may wish, also, to see an ear, nose, and throat (ENT) specialist. The opposite situation can also be true, where an infected tooth is the cause of sinus pain.

Angina and myocardial infarction

Heart pain can be referred to the teeth. Nitroglycerine often relieves angina pain. If a heart attack (myocardial infarction) is suspected, call 911 and take aspirin if acceptable.

Middle ear infection

A middle ear infection, which is also called acute otitis media, can send pain to the teeth. This should be ruled out to prevent unnecessary dental treatment.

Malignancy

Cancer can refer pain to the teeth and must be ruled out if a dental origin is unclear.

Headache disorders

Many different types of headaches can refer pain to the teeth. This is particularly true with cluster headaches.

Herpes

Oral herpes and shingles breakouts are notorious for leading to tooth pain both during and a long time after the herpes episode.

Trigeminal neuralgia

Trigeminal neuralgia is a neuropathic pain affecting the trigeminal facial nerve that can come on suddenly and reoccur. This disease can cause tooth pain.

Takeaway

If you have oral pain, there can be various causes to consider. This is especially true if your dentist does a procedure like a root canal to alleviate the pain and the nature of the pain does not change or disappear. Make sure you consider: muscular pain; inflammation of the nerves due to viral, bacterial, chemical, or traumatic causes; salivary gland infection or blockage; damage to your neck (cervical) nerves; pressure on your mental nerve due to jaw resorption; blood vessel and associated nerve dysfunction; and pain of psychological origin, including Munchausen syndrome.

Eighteen

Emergencies & Tooth Trauma

Time matters when emergencies occur. Sudden damage to your teeth can happen anywhere and at any time. Being prepared in advance for this unexpected incident requires knowing just a few things.

The information in this chapter is based on my understanding of the new multi-country accepted treatment standards and is written as if I was giving directions to a dental student (not for the general public to act upon). This is what you should expect from a dentist and not for you to do on your own. Diagrams have been included to rapidly identify the trauma type. Every emergency is different, and this chapter is provided as information only and should not be considered a substitute for obtaining immediate care by a qualified dentist or physician.

Types of Tooth Trauma

Adult tooth knocked out

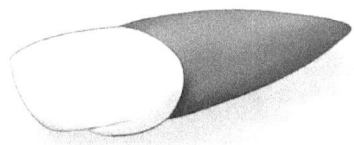

Figure 18.1. An adult tooth that has been knocked out of the mouth.

If an entire adult tooth is knocked out of your mouth, do not touch the root (the part of the tooth that is normally under the gums). Try to only touch the crown of the tooth (the part that is normally visible when you smile). You want to immediately rinse off any dirt and then push the tooth back into the hole (socket) where it came from, despite any bleeding.

Bite on a clean piece of cloth and go to the dentist as soon as possible. If you cannot put the tooth back in, then put it in milk or in the commonly available Save-A-Tooth® 24-hour preservation kit and go to the dentist immediately. Soaking the tooth in regular tap water will destroy the skin tissues that are attached to the root. A quick rinse in tap water to remove dirt is not a problem but soaking the tooth in tap water is a problem. Tissues still on the root need to be alive to reattach the tooth properly to the jaw.

The prognosis is great for teeth that have been knocked out if they are placed back in the socket within twenty minutes. The prognosis is good for teeth replaced within sixty minutes. The prognosis is much worse after sixty minutes.

Because there will be some bacteria remaining on the root, it may be prudent for the injured person to take amoxicillin or penicillin to help prevent localized infection. In cases of amoxicillin or penicillin allergy, doxycycline can be the best choice for anybody over age twelve. (Doxycycline stains the growing teeth permanently in children twelve years and under.)

On occasion, your dentist may need to hold the injured tooth in its natural position. In that case, a flexible wire splint can be cemented to the injured tooth and the adjacent teeth for two to four weeks.

If a completely knocked-out tooth has been reimplanted into the socket, a dentist may elect to do root canal therapy with calcium hydroxide (a tissue-compatible material that has a hard tissue inducing effect) at seven to ten days. This decision must be made by the dentist based on a combination of several clinical factors.

Baby tooth knocked out

If a baby tooth is knocked out, just leave it out. Replacing it back into the socket can damage the adult tooth underneath, which has not yet erupted and can still be soft. Additionally, if you put a baby tooth back in the socket, it will often fall out quickly because a baby tooth has short roots and the child will play with the tooth with their tongue. The child can accidentally choke on the loose tooth and breathe the tooth into his or her lungs. It will mean a trip to the emergency room if this happens.

You should take the child to the dentist in the next few days after a baby tooth is knocked out. The dentist may need to place a device to hold the empty space open so permanent teeth will still have room to erupt where the baby tooth is missing. This is particularly true for back teeth.

Cut lip or tongue

If a person has a tooth knocked out and also suffers a cut lip or tongue, you still should deal with the tooth first. This is because the odds are good that the tooth will survive if the tooth is replaced into the socket within twenty minutes. The soft tissue damage of a cut lip or tongue rarely has such a critical time requirement unless a large blood vessel is cut and the lip or tongue is pumping out life-threatening amounts of blood. If so, apply pressure and call an ambulance.

Tooth partially knocked out

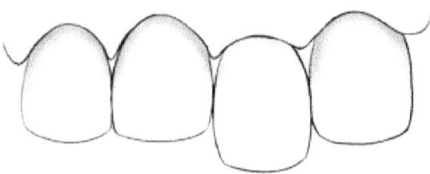

Figure 18.2. A tooth only partially knocked out.

If the injured tooth was never fully knocked out of the mouth and a dentist was present at the scene, they would immediately push the tooth back into its original position, have the patient bite on a clean cloth, and go to the office to possibly stabilize the tooth with an acrylic bond. The sooner this is accomplished, the better, because you do not want a blood clot forming at the bottom of the socket preventing the tooth from being moved back into position. See the dentist immediately, as this is an emergency. If the tooth is only a little loose due to the injury, bite on a clean cloth and see the dentist as soon as possible.

Injury pushes the tooth deeper into the jawbone

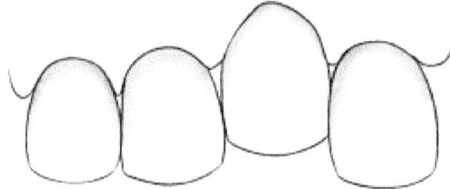

Figure 18.3. A tooth jammed deeper into the jawbone.

If the tooth has been jammed deeper into the jawbone due to the injury, do not move the tooth. Luckily, when a tooth has been shoved deeper into the jaw, many teeth will re-erupt naturally back to the original ideal position. Have the person bite on a clean cloth and see a dentist ASAP. It is important to have a dentist evaluate this tooth initially and again in two weeks, then every three months.

Natural crown breaks off

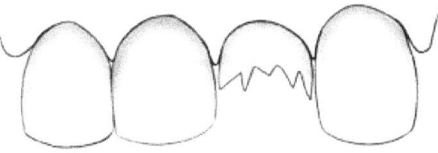

Figure 18.4. A natural crown is snapped off.

If the natural tooth's crown is broken off, but the tooth's root remains in the mouth, keep the piece of the tooth that was broken off moist in water (a dry tooth changes color), and bring it to the dentist. This will assist the dentist to make a good color and shape choice for a replacement crown or filling. Occasionally the broken piece can even be cemented back onto the tooth.

Broken jaw

If the entire jawbone is broken or the jawbone no longer lines up, you need go to a medical emergency room immediately.

Artificial crown falls off or is knocked off

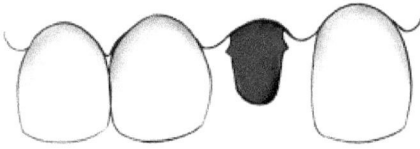

Figure 18.5. An artificial crown comes off.

Do not try to put the artificial crown back in the mouth. It is rarely a problem to wait a few days to have your dentist fix the tooth. Do not try to replace the artificial crown onto the tooth until a dentist can cement it on properly. This reduces the risk of swallowing or aspirating the crown into your lungs if it slides off again. There are many instances where a crown has been slid back onto the tooth just for esthetics and then fell out and was aspirated into the lungs. If a crown gets in your lungs, it means you must go to the emergency room.

It is particularly foolish to slide a loose crown onto a tooth or use a do-it-yourself pharmacy tooth glue kit to improve your esthetics temporarily. I hope you will consider these options even more ill-advised when I tell you there are plenty of instances when perfect front teeth are knocked out by an emergency room physician or surgeon trying to get a crown out of someone's lungs. This risk of additional broken teeth is so great it is included on the ER physician's medical consent forms.

Follow-Up Visits

After the initial dental visit for the trauma, five follow-up dental visits are usually recommended at the following intervals: seven-to-ten days; four weeks; three months; six months; and at a year after the injury.

Different problems can arise at these various time intervals, and this follow-up schedule should be adhered to. Anytime there is tooth trauma, a root canal or extraction may eventually be needed.

Nineteen

How to Choose a Dentist

The average family in the United States moves to a different neighborhood, city, or state every six years. This means most of us need to choose new health care practitioners fairly often. Knowing what sources to trust can help you with this choice. Like other businesses, some dental practices can incentivize patients to leave good reviews and to take down bad reviews. Most users posting dental office reviews are not knowledgeable about the quality of the technical aspects of the dentistry they are commenting on. I have seen five-star reviews posted for treatment performed that was serious malpractice. The procedure didn't hurt, so the patient was happy.

In addition to assuring you are getting quality dental work, you also want to choose a dentist carefully to avoid being a victim of fraud. According to the National Health Care Anti-Fraud Association, approximately $12.5 billion is lost to dental fraud and abuse each year.

Understanding the essential facts about dentistry explained in this book are crucial to maximizing your dental health. The concepts in this chapter will help you find an excellent dentist and avoid excessive treatment and unexpected, poor results.

"First, Do No Harm"

"First, do no harm" is a principle that defines an important obligation of health care providers. This is why health education is entirely directed at teaching how

to provide the best possible care. Newly graduated dentists come out of school after four years of learning how to accurately diagnose and perform the best treatment for each given diagnosis. The philosophy of keeping the patient's interests before financial gain is the basis for everything that is taught in dental school and has historically guided dentists' care in their own private practices for over 100 years. Recently, however, situations have changed. Student loan debt has exploded to an average of over $280,000.00 and fewer new dentists can afford to open up private offices of their own. Many new dentists end up working under the direction of large corporations. The corporate philosophy can redirect the dentist's focus on what is good for the patient toward what is good for the corporation's bottom line.

Decades ago, *Consumer Reports*® started protecting the public by nearly single-handedly reporting on dangerous and unreliable cars. This improved the safety and quality of our automobiles. And more recently *Consumer Reports*®, in their September 2022 issue, featured an article headlined "Do You Really Need That Root Canal, Crown, or Implant?" The report discusses dentistry in general, but includes this warning: "For example, private equity-owned dental service organizations may encourage some dentists to sell people unnecessary treatments to maximize profits."

A New Corporate Mantra?

Today, *"Maximize daily production and profit"* can be a mantra of dental corporations. Corporate dental chains and private equity owned dental service organizations (DSOs) are a major provider of dental care (the DSO market size is around 100 billion dollars).

Corporate dental chains and private equity dental service organizations are companies that own or manage dental offices and establish protocols to make maximum profit.

These corporate dental chains and private equity dental service organizations owned by large corporations or hedge funds have been rapidly opening multiple dental practices. They obtain patients by massive advertising efforts.

One of the largest dental chains currently in business settled a lawsuit with the Massachusetts Attorney General's Office for $3.5 million over deceptive advertising methods according to a 2023 press release from the Massachusetts

Office of the Attorney General. The lawsuit alleged the corporate dental organization "engaged in a multi-faceted scheme to deceive consumers into purchasing dental services…" and sent consumers to collections over bills for services it advertised as "free." Previously, in 2014, the same chain was required to pay almost $1 million in a settlement of a lawsuit with Massachusetts also alleging deceptive advertising and marketing practices. The plaintiffs in that case claimed the massive dental chain lured them with promises of free x-rays or exams and low-cost treatment, then charged them anyway, and/or pressured them into other treatment. The company's corporate revenue is approaching a billion dollars a year and they are in business across the United States.

These dental corporations continue to thrive despite large settlements for several reasons. One reason is because the public is not aware of these judgments. Another reason is these corporations are extremely rich and powerful. Solo practitioners cannot survive million-dollar judgments, but corporate dental groups and DSOs are profitable enough to survive large judgments and continue to thrive.

Another reason corporations thrive is because the United States government usually battles health care fraud with the civil justice system, rather than with the criminal justice system, to speed up court proceedings and reduce government legal costs. The civil system almost never forces defendants to acknowledge their guilt and notify patients of their fraud. This minimizes the effect of the punishment and how many members of the public learn of the seriousness of these transgressions.

A corporation's directors are legally beholden to doing what is best for the stockholders, not for any individual patient or employee. Doctors and dentists are obligated to provide for the best interest of the patient. Thus, there is an inherent conflict when a dentist is employed by a corporate dental chain or a private equity-owned dental service organization. Pressure from your employer is hard to ignore.

Legal disciplinary actions by state boards of dental examiners are almost exclusively against individual dentists, not the corporations that manage or own the practices. One reason for this is because the employee dentist usually must acknowledge in their initial contract that all treatment decisions are entirely up to the employee dentist and the corporation is not to be held liable for their treatment decisions. This contract is signed and agreed to before the employee dentist actually experiences the production pressures and difficulties in obtaining and examining daily billing records as we discuss in this chapter.

In my anecdotal experience I have never talked to a dentist working for a large corporate dental chain that did not receive directions and input from their corporate management that attempted to influence the treatment choices and pressure the dentist by giving feedback such as, "You need to do more crowns instead of fillings," or other similarly coercive comments to encourage overtreatment. This attempt to influence the dentist to do more production is specifically illegal in most states if the provider of the coercion is not a dentist. For instance, in Texas, the Texas Administrative Code, Section 251.003, subsection (a) 9, states you are practicing dentistry (and must be a licensed dentist) if you attempt to control or influence a dentist's diagnosis or treatment of a dental disease.

Dental malpractice is an additional troublesome issue. Ninety-nine percent of medical and dental education revolves around learning how to treat disease as perfectly as possible. When doctors and dentists make errors in the provision of health care, they are personally, professionally, and criminally held accountable by the legal system and state boards.

When corporate dental chains and DSOs get named in dental malpractice lawsuits, however, the company's shareholders and executives are often not held legally or criminally responsible for damaging people's health. They are protected by something called the corporate veil. You can search for the list of disciplinary actions by any state's board of dental examiners. You will find a list of offending individual dentists, often working for large dental groups, but almost never are these corporate dental chains listed or punished for malpractice.

Dentists can be hired as employees, associate dentists, partial owners, or independent contractors. For simplicity, I will call them all employee dentists.

Questionable billing

The U.S. Government investigations found large dental chains were major contributors to questionable billing for Medicaid pediatric dental services in several states:

- The U.S. Office of Inspector General, Department of Health & Human Services, in an Office of Evaluations and Inspections report (OEI-02-14-00480) for California determined: "A concentration of providers with questionable billing in chains raises concerns that these chains are encouraging their providers to perform unnecessary procedures to illegally increase profits."

- Investigating Indiana, the U.S. Office of Inspector General in a report (OEI-02-14-00250) reported, "Notably, two thirds of the general dentists with questionable billing worked for four dental chains in Indiana. Three of these chains have been the subject of Federal and State investigations. A concentration of such providers in chains raises concerns that these chains may be encouraging their providers to perform unnecessary procedures to increase profits."

- In New York (OEI-02-12-00330), of the dentists identified with questionable billing, the U.S. Office of Inspector General found the following: "Additionally, almost a third of the general dentists were associated with a single dental chain that had settled lawsuits for providing services that were medically unnecessary or failed to meet professionally recognized standard of care to children."

The reports above concerned dental treatment on children. Most of these large group dental practices still exist. Read these cases and decide on your own if you want to support these dental chains.

Staff dedication is to who pays them

You want the staff to be paid directly by the dentist, so they are motivated to help the dentist do their best work. It is rare to find a staff completely dedicated to helping the dentist provide the best possible patient care if a corporation, not the dentist, is in control of their employment and signs their paychecks.

Pressure to work too quickly

There can be pressure by the corporation and staff to produce as much as possible each day. Pressure to work more quickly than is comfortable for the employee dentist can clearly result in a reduction in quality. Corporate dental chains often pay their dentists as little as possible per procedure. I have seen hundreds of cases where the corporate practice dentist has recently done a crown or filling and never removed all of the decay since removing all of the decay properly would take two or three times longer to complete the same procedure. This means the remaining decay will get worse rapidly and the patient will lose the tooth or need a root canal and more treatment. They can make the employee dentists do the advertised "free" dental exams without pay. This adds more pressure to work as fast as possible. Excellent dentistry is accomplished by taking the time to double-check each step and look at the tooth from every angle. It is also accomplished by doing a careful comprehensive exam and creating a complete set of records when initially seeing a patient rather than doing a quick, cheap exam. You can search Glassdoor.com and other employment sites to find comments by dentists who work for dental offices you may be considering.

Pressures to do it all

A dentist may only want to do the procedures they are comfortable and competent at performing. Dentists in corporate dental chains can receive pressure to do nearly every dental procedure. This includes procedures that they may not be comfortable performing and would normally send to a specialist in root canals, periodontology, orthodontics, or oral surgery. If the same dentist worked outside of this high-pressure environment, that dentist would be more likely to refer patients to a specialist for complex procedures. Not referring patients to appropriate specialists can result in poorer work, misdiagnoses, failed procedures, and possibly lost teeth. The patient is usually not aware of this difference in quality until months or years later. Furthermore, if the corporate dental office or DSO has its own in-house specialist, the in-house specialist can be under the same kind of production pressures to work quickly. A dentist in their own private practice is mostly concerned with their long-term reputation and the excellence of their work rather than the one-time day's profit.

Be knowledgeable about social media

The internet and social media are great and powerful resources. But don't trust social media or reviews as your sole source for third-party endorsements. When people search for a dentist online, the most likely offices to show up first are those that can afford a professionally optimized website and pay the highest bids per click to their website.

The dental offices with the most money to spend are often the large corporations. In addition, some dental chains can have professional teams with persuasive scripts and various inducements to motivate angry reviewers to remove poor ratings. This diminishes the value of the rating system and harms the ability of the general public to make properly informed judgments.

Hiding their ownership

Despite their efforts, some dental offices cannot convince the angriest of dental patients to remove their ratings online and eventually it can be seen they have bad reputations. Because they cannot fully control all of the worst reviews on social media nor prevent people from seeing their lawsuits in the news, some dental chains have renamed and established new dental practices hiding the truth of their ownership. If they had good reputations, they would be proud of their ownership and not hide behind some other name.

The United States Attorney's Office Central District of Illinois issued a press release headlined, "Illinois Dental Management Company to Pay $3 Million To Settle Allegations of Improper Billing, Dentist Registration." The company named in this release has approximately 1,000 offices and is now opening more dental offices with different catchy names obscuring who owns and manages these offices. They paid the fine and stayed in business.

How to identify who owns a dental office

You must find out who *owns or manages* the dental practice, not just the name of the possibly temporary dentist working there. The true ownership and license must be registered with state and local government offices and the U.S. Beneficial Ownership Registration Registry. A surefire way to determine if it is a corporation that owns the practice is to look for names on brochures or on business cards or on the bottom of website pages that differ from the name of the dentist who is treating you. This occurs because the dentists are often temporary and reprinting all stationary every time there is a new dentist is an expense a corporation wants to avoid. Also check if their email address ends in a corporate chain website address. Corporations often don't have the website biography of the actual dentist working in the practice since they may see them as temporary employees. Having a dentist's bio on the website is not a green flag, but the absence of one is a red flag.

Why do Dentists Work for these Employers?

Consider the following facts: 1) a large number of dentists in the United States are **foreign nationals**; 2) the average dental student in the United States comes out of school with **$312,000.00 in student debt**. These two groups of dentists have limited options. Many foreign national dentists need their employer to sponsor them or they lose their green cards and must leave the United States. New graduates with $280,000.00 in student debt are limited in their ability to get bank loans and open a private practice. The corporate dental chains and DSOs often hire these new graduates and foreign nationals.

Be Wary of these Issues in Dental Offices

Upcoding

Upcoding occurs when the office changes the correct treatment code of a service to one that allows a larger amount to be billed. Upcoding simple extractions to surgical extractions, for example, is extremely common in any dental office where the main objective is making money as quickly as possible. (Insurance code D7140 is the code for a simple extraction. D7210 is the code for a more complex surgical extraction where the crown and the root break during the extraction and both pieces are removed.) I have heard of one multi-state group practice found in the Southern States where this upcoding fraud is a habit. A surgical extraction fee is much higher than a simple extraction. This makes the bill over 50% higher.

The Texas Health and Human Services Office of Inspector General recently found another common upcoding fraud is dental sealants billed as restorations.

If you are concerned about proper dental billing, the descriptions of every dental insurance code are found in a book called, *"Current Dental Terminology®® (CDT®)."* More elaborate descriptions are found in the book *"CDT Coding Companion®."*

Pressure on the dentist by the staff

If the employee dentist working in some private practices or corporate chains does not produce or upsell adequately, then the staff members do not get bonuses. A production and bonus-oriented staff can influence the dentist to comply with the maximum profit mantra in different ways. For example: the staff can cause the dentist pain by overbooking the schedule, not ordering requested preferred instruments and supplies, and ignoring instructions. The employee dentist is not in charge of hiring and firing the uncooperative employees. Additionally, corporate dental chains and DSOs often require employee dentists to sign long-period agreements before the dentists experience the actual working conditions. The employee dentist must continue to work with staff that can pressure the dentist to finish dental procedures as quickly as possible rather than taking the extra time that excellent dentistry requires.

Professionally created sales techniques

For years large dental chains have developed effective sales and closing techniques to maximize profit. Large dental chains often hire office staff members from high pressure sales backgrounds to present these closing sales pitches to patients. Some multi-location dental offices state in their ads for hiring front office employees that they are looking for sales backgrounds, not dental or medical backgrounds. These staff members are placed in positions to present treatment plans and fees to patients. Staff members hired from sales backgrounds are accustomed to trying to obtain the largest purchase possible from each customer. It is possible the front desk staff's main goal is to pressure you toward a maximum purchase commitment, rather than looking out for your dental and financial health. Companies that teach sales and effective closing techniques are starting to market to all dentists. Make sure to be aware that this kind of sales pressure is starting to be more prevalent in many dental offices, not just corporations.

Be wary of extensive same-day treatment

When you go in for a routine dental exam and the dentist presents the treatment plan, they may wish to start as many procedures as possible immediately. There are several problems with an extensive "same-day treatment" approach for you as a patient:

- You do not have the opportunity to evaluate and learn about the alternative treatments.

- You cannot compare fees for the procedures.

- You do not have the opportunity to get a second opinion.

- The proper length of time for the appointment is probably not already built into the schedule. This means that the dentist or the hygienist may be rushed to finish the procedure before the next patient. This is particularly dangerous to your health when the dental hygienist attempts to do four quadrants of root planing, or even two, in a normal simple cleaning appointment time slot.

The risks to the patient who agrees to same-day treatment are particularly acute when services are provided as part of a bundled treatment plan without individual fees detailed.

Bundled treatment presentations

Some national dental chains and some private practices instruct their office staff not to provide patients with a complete breakdown of procedures with associated fees. Dental practices that provide a bundled treatment price, rather than a specific breakdown of each planned procedure and associated fees, should be a cause for concern. This arrangement can lead to unexpected payment issues for you when insurance companies refuse to pay for questionable treatment fees. For instance, particular per-tooth medications or medications used in the process of cleaning teeth are often not paid for by insurance companies and you are left paying unexpected fees. Some large practices combine minimal value services with an insurance company negotiated low-priced root planing fee. The insurance pays the low root planing fee, but you must pay the remaining extra fees for the minimally valuable, expensive add-on treatments.

Bundling the fees and treatments also make it difficult to know if some procedures were performed. In addition, you cannot figure out how much they are charging for standard procedures so you cannot compare the price of their treatment with costs at other providers. You might want to run in the other direction when you see this tactic used for anything other than complex full mouth rehabilitation treatment involving several implants and prosthetics.

There is no harm in getting a second opinion if you feel there are too many procedures recommended in a lump sum presentation. This is especially true if no one has shown you the issues in your own mouth. It is important to most people to have a list of what procedures are needed, their cost, and which are critical to have done first. Having a list of procedures allows budgeting and coordinating the use of your benefits and out of pocket expenses.

Unbundling

Unbundling is separately billing the component parts of a dental procedure, rather than billing the single code for the procedure. This fraudulently allows the office to bill for a cumulative charge that is higher than that assigned to a proper procedure code. For instance, a billing code for a gingival flap procedure includes root planing done at the same time. It is unbundling if you are billed separately for both root planing and a gingival flap procedure done in the same area at the same time.

Replacing old work

Avoid dentists who advise you to have your fillings replaced just because the average filling of that type is replaced at "X" number of years. If a dentist says this, run the other way to a different dentist. Replacing fillings just because they are "so many years old" leads to more tooth structure being removed and increases your eventual risk of tooth loss over time. Make sure the dentist can show you a defect in the filling rather than just says this tooth is older than "X" number of years, so they are going to replace it.

Revolving door

You do not want to go to a corporate or private dental office where dentists do not stay for many years. Check how long your dentist has been in that practice. A reason why dentists leave practices is because they are concerned about their legal and malpractice liability. One common example is: employee dentists in large group practices can have very little access to and control over what treatment code is being charged for when a second party is submitting billing. The employee dentist is still liable. Even where access is given, a daily fight to review every procedure at the end of each day does not promote a comfortable work environment. In addition, if one dentist commits malpractice, every dentist who has seen that patient, or supervised the hygienist when they saw the patient, will be named a in a lawsuit despite their lack of culpability. Other examples of extra risks to employee dentists are too numerous to enumerate here.

Unnecessary treatment

Unfortunately, suggesting unnecessary treatment is becoming more common. Patients needing minor treatment such as a new filling might be told they need a crown instead. A good dentist will be happy to show you the area of concern in a photo, x-ray, or mirror. It is important that you ask to see the problem.

Some dental practices will administer expensive saliva tests to each patient saying they are for evaluating bacteria that cause periodontal disease and cavities. Then they will use the test results in patient treatment planning. However, these tests often have an unacceptable amount of false positive and negative results making them untrustworthy. The FDA checks for efficacy and trustworthiness of these tests. I would check that the suggested saliva test is FDA-approved before undergoing and paying for one.

Some practices are using Cone Beam CT scans because they made a large monetary investment in the machine and want to recoup the cost. Patients are charged hundreds of dollars for Cone Beam CT scans and exposed to much higher doses of radiation than traditional panoramic and dental x-rays. These should rarely be an initial new patient scanning device. This is particularly true for children because they are highly sensitive to radiation. I believe Cone Beam CT scans should be limited to specific issues and complex cases such as those for TMJ disorders, pathology, complex orthodontics, dental implants, complex endodontics, and extractions.

Unlicensed staff performing dental procedures

Having unlicensed staff members doing dental cleanings and supervising laughing gas administration is illegal and dangerous. This is a common problem. Scaling and root planing can only be done by a licensed hygienist or dentist. Separate credentials are required to supervise a patient while under nitrous oxide sedation. Licenses for these procedures are maintained and updated by the respective dental state boards and should be posted at the dental office.

Quotas

Once seen mostly in corporate offices, today many private dental offices set a daily officewide and sometimes per patient production quota. Offices are doing this after taking classes on maximizing profits. These offices and dental chains have daily meetings with staff, hygienists, and employee dentists, where the manager reviews production of the previous day and whether the office, hygienist, or the dentist met their daily numbers. They also present the production numbers expected for the current day. The whole office is usually concerned they could be fired—or not make bonuses—if they do not meet quotas. The staff can then put pressure on the dentist to produce more on each patient and work more quickly. I have recently seen some offices offer a below average base pay for dental hygienists but provide extra pay if they upsell products or services. These extras are rarely as valuable as providing you with the careful root planing or cleanings you came in for.

Health care should be based on meeting the needs of the patient, and not on finding something expensive to do each day. Becoming a pawn of this system makes no sense for any reasonable patient to accept. The quota pressure means patients may be urged to accept unnecessary and expensive work.

When your dentist doesn't tell you why you need X, Y, and Z treatment, but rather a front desk employee comes over and gives you a list of things you need, that can be problematic. Your dentist should be able to explain to you and show you any of the dental issues you have. Don't be afraid to ask questions and request to see the cavity or defect they are suggesting needs treatment.

Which Dentist to Choose?

There are several advantages to choosing a local, patient-focused dentist who is committed to building a private practice.

Committed to your local community

Dentists that *live and permanently practice in your local area* rather than continually change their office of employment are motivated to do their very best work and not overcharge you. They know they are likely to see their patients at the grocery store, kids' school events, and community gatherings. These locally established dentists rely heavily on word-of-mouth promotion for their business and protect their reputations. They are clearly planning for the long haul.

Keeps reliable staff

A good dentist knows that *keeping and rewarding experienced, reliable staff* makes their dental work better and safer. A staff that has longevity will become well-acquainted with the patients. Because a long-term staff member has repeatedly reviewed, discussed, and updated your health history, fewer medical issues that can impact your treatment and health are overlooked. Continually looking for the least expensive staff is not a hallmark of a good dental practice.

Knows your dental history

A good dentist who treats you over a number of years knows your habits and dental treatment history. If you see the same dentist, then fillings can sometimes be repaired or patched, and an entirely new filling is not needed. If your treating dentist performed the original filling and noticed over time that it has developed a small defect, they can be confident that all the decay was previously removed because they did the filling. The advantage of keeping most of the original filling is that far less tooth structure needs to be removed, which helps you keep your teeth over a lifetime.

If you go to a different dentist who does not know the quality of the work of the previous dentist that did the filling, a completely new filling is often done. This is to make sure the deepest area is free of decay because x-rays often do not show decay immediately underneath a dental filling.

It is important to realize every time a filling or crown is replaced, more tooth is being removed. This means you are that much closer to eventually losing the tooth because there is not enough tooth structure left to resist biting forces.

When the dentist knows you and is comfortable that you are going to return to them in six months to a year, they can watch small areas of demineralization or tiny, early cavities and have you attempt to regenerate the enamel with fluoride and special oral hygiene efforts. If the dentist is a temporary employee and likely to never see you again, they will feel motivated to treat every small defect, even those small surface areas that may remineralize with directed good oral hygiene.

Refers to specialists

A dentist committed to providing the best treatment for their patients *decides on the procedures they are best at and will refer to specialists for more complex issues.* The procedures they feel less competent doing are referred to a network of specialists they are confident in.

Minimizing radiation

You can minimize radiation by staying at one office. This is because transfers of x-rays to other offices often are inadequate, incomplete, and not usually transferred at full resolution. So, x-rays end up being retaken. When diagnosing and treating dental disease, the amount of radiation should always follow the guiding principle of ALARA, "as low as reasonably achievable."

Second opinions

A good dentist is not afraid of a patient getting a second opinion, since a good diagnosis is often indisputable. Different treatment approaches to fix a particular diagnosis can vary, but the diagnosis should be verifiable. Most people have situations that should be watched but may never need treatment. An unethical or pressured dentist can take advantage of any gray area of diagnosis to maximize immediate production.

Do not be reluctant to get a second opinion. Intuition exists for a reason. If you feel uncomfortable or the treatment plan does not seem right, go get a second opinion. Printed x-rays on paper can be of minimal value and will usually need to be retaken. E-mailed x-rays have some limitations but are more likely to be acceptable to a different dentist, especially if sent at full resolution.

Tell the second opinion office you want a complete exam and treatment plan. To get the most information, do not show the new office the previous treatment plan. Even an extensive second opinion examination should be inexpensive compared to treatment. You can compare the two treatment plans and examine them for the care taken, completeness of evaluation, and if overtreatment planning seems likely. The section on the comprehensive exam later in this chapter explains what should be included. Studies show that half of dental patients who get a second opinion end up changing their course of treatment.

You will almost always benefit from a second opinion and either dentist will undoubtedly be happy with your decision to choose them. Being chosen after a second opinion is a compliment to them and their staff.

Ask a periodontist for a referral to a general dentist

Seeing or calling a periodontal specialist can help you choose an excellent dentist. Poor dentistry magnifies the speed at which gum disease progresses because badly fitting fillings and crowns trap and hold bacteria that cause gum disease. Even a tenth of a millimeter defect on a filling or crown traps millions of bacteria and causes a red area of inflamed gum tissue. Periodontists hate it when poor dentistry is done after their efforts to control the gum disease is completed. I have never seen a periodontist working in their own private practice refer patients to a bad dentist. The easiest way to find a good dentist is to ask a periodontist not financially associated with a group practice for a recommendation for a dentist.

My Opinion: Is Dental "Insurance" Really Insurance?

Dental insurance companies can have a maximum allowance of $1,000 to $2,000 per year. This is often the same yearly maximum paid out forty years ago! The plan may limit the number of procedures allowed per year or per tooth, have a waiting period, or may only pay 50% of their own low fee schedule instead of the dentist's normal fee schedule.

Obviously, the failure to increase annual amounts of insurance policy payouts to match inflation over decades means increased profits for dental insurance companies. The proportion of dental insurance companies' income enriching their executives and stockholders compared to the proportion going to actual dental treatment has risen to extreme levels.

Some states are trying to pass laws that would force dental insurance companies to spend a more reasonable percentage of their monthly premiums on patient care. In November 2022, Massachusetts passed a law that requires dental insurance carriers to spend at least 83% of their premiums on patient care.

To obtain better dental insurance, we should all suggest to our own state legislators that they enact laws like the one Massachusetts passed.

There are advantages to choosing a dentist who does not take dental insurance. A dentist that does not carry dental insurance can have less overhead, so their fees can be lower. In fact, one of the largest recent increases of dental office expenses is the cost of eligibility and benefit verification for patients, which increased by 15% to $2.1 billion in 2023. Instead of your money going towards treatment, you are paying for verification software and/or a dedicated dental staff specialist to sit on the phone waiting on hold for an insurance person to eventually come to the phone and provide or clarify information. Even with you paying for this effort and expense, I have seen where the insurance company denies that the conversation ever happened even when identified by the name of the insurance employee and the conversation record number. This is another hidden waste of your money when you or your employer buy dental insurance. Dentists who do not accept dental insurance can give discounts to patients in financial need. In my experience with over 1000 dentists, they are a particularly compassionate group of people interested in helping others with their healthcare. Most are generous with providing extra procedures at no cost or providing discounts unless they are employed by corporations that are judging their daily production or have insurance companies that limit their discounting abilities. Dentists who are in-network insurance providers cannot allow reduced fees. If a dentist is an in-network provider of an insurance plan and the dentist starts discounting fees off the insurance contracted amount to help patients in financial distress, the dentist will be penalized severely. Dental insurance contracts usually say the discounted fee given to some patients must be established as a new contracted amount for everyone. Then they can force the dentist to refund to the insurance company the discounted amount. This demand that dentists repay the insurance companies can include procedures done up to six years in the past on every previous patient. A large amount of the dues paid by members of the American Dental Association and the Academy of General Dentistry are used to lobby legislatures to allow dentists to give discounts to patients despite insurance rules. This alone is a good reason to seek out dentists that belong to these two associations.

Dental insurance is a minor assistance for a small amount of treatment each year. If you have lots of dental work to do, you may be better off going to a dentist who does not take dental insurance and is not prohibited from giving you a fee reduction.

Insurance companies have begun leasing out dental practice services to other provider insurance networks by default. This is done without the express consent of the dentist that only agreed to be a provider on the first insurance plan. This can result in a less than expected insurance payment only realized after the insurance settles. This leaves the patient with a higher amount to pay than expected. Dental insurance companies have also recently started paying dentists by credit cards without their consent. This comes with serious fees and reduces dentists' income which ultimately results in increased costs to patients.

Many experts have noted that dental insurance companies have developed too much power and are hurting consumers and dentists. The proof of this is seen in recent settlements against a large insurance company of $2.67 billion to its subscribers and a separate settlement of $2.8 billion to its providers. States such as Oregon and California are fighting to protect the consumer and the dentists from these profit grabs by insurance companies.

Dental financing programs and cards

There are many dental financing programs and medical credit cards to allow you to get dental treatment performed and make an interest-free payment each month for twelve months or longer. The dentist offers these plans because the finance company pays the dentist 80% to 90% of the fee immediately and the financing company assumes responsibility to collect the fee from the patient. This is a convenient way to get work done that makes both the patient and the dentist happy. These plans can be convenient to use if you are careful.

If you elect this method of financing, you must make sure that you can pay it off before the time limit. If you don't, you will get an immediate bill for the accumulated deferred interest. Since the credit company cannot repossess your dental work, if you buy dental work with this type of credit, they can come after valuable assets you own, sometimes including your home. Be sure the amount due is an amount you can afford to pay each month and will be able to pay off before the interest escalation clause comes into effect.

On May 4, 2023, the U.S. White House administration cautioned Americans about using these financing devices to pay for medical and dental bills. They are concerned they may lead to bankruptcy for too many people. In addition, United States Senator Elizabeth Warren also warned in 2023 that the

Consumer Financial Protection Bureau should take action to protect patients from these potentially risky programs.

Here is What to Expect from a Good Dentist

Most of this book is dedicated to explaining procedures and providing an understanding of the risks and benefit of each treatment. The potential problems we discussed can usually be avoided by seeing a good dentist. You can tell you are seeing a good dentist if you experience the kinds of services described below.

The comprehensive exam

A comprehensive exam should be done the first time you visit a new dentist. If it is done in only fifteen minutes, critical issues like measurements for gum disease or an oral cancer examination are likely to have been overlooked. A comprehensive exam for adults should include the following components:

- *X-rays clearly showing the contact between the teeth.* These x-rays often need to be done every six to eighteen months if you have already experienced cavities and every twenty-four to thirty-six months if you have not had cavities.

- *X-rays showing the root tips of every tooth.* These periapical or panoramic x-rays should be taken approximately every two to four years. A complete set of x-rays showing the root tips of every tooth is your best insurance against your dentist missing infections. The x-rays showing root tips can also help the dentist detect cancer in the jawbone and serious infections that can spread to your bloodstream and your brain.

- *A complete periodontal exam.* This exam includes taking at least six pocket depth measurements on *each* tooth. Recession, bleeding, and tissue type should also be recorded. Tell them in advance that you would like a copy of your periodontal exam for your health records; this will make it far more likely that an accurate exam is done. Never forget that periodontal disease is the main cause of adults losing their teeth. A careful evaluation of your gum disease status can take at least ten to thirty minutes of the full exam time but is critical to your health.

- *An oral cancer exam.* This should include pulling the tongue to the left and right sides since oral cancer often exists on the sides of the tongue. It should also include feeling the muscles and spaces around your mouth.

- *An examination of each tooth.* The dentist should carefully examine all the teeth for cavities and wear. An examination of the x-rays can be done simultaneously.

- *A sleep apnea analysis.* Since 2017, this is suggested as an important part of a dental exam.

- *A temporomandibular joint exam.* Your jaw joints should be evaluated for clicking pain and muscular discomfort.

- *A bite analysis.* The way your jaws meet each other and how the teeth hit each other can influence your treatment.

- *An oral history of your dental care.* A discussion of your habits, oral hygiene, and past medical and dental treatments can be very important.

Although a careful exam takes time, it is the least expensive procedure in per-hour costs and the most important part of your dental treatment. Invest in a careful exam. It will benefit you in many ways.

A comprehensive exam can allow your dentist to properly develop a sequence of treatment based on health risks, expense, and your personal preferences. A careful exam defines the necessary work needed immediately versus at some time in the future and avoids putting money into teeth that may be lost soon. It also allows you and your dentist to plan for a more proactive approach to do your future treatment when it fits your schedule and wallet. Without a comprehensive exam, you will be playing Whack-a-mole with your teeth and your finances.

The consultation

Your dentist should tell you about the risks, benefits, and alternatives of any proposed treatment.

If you have a complex situation and need to decide between extracting or restoring a tooth, the dentist should present multiple options. If your dentist suggests keeping the tooth, it may be prudent to go with their suggestion.

Keeping a tooth with periodontal disease could involve surgery and grafting. This may sound daunting and extracting the tooth and placing an implant may sound simpler and easier. Recent scientific research suggests many teeth, including many periodontally diseased teeth, will often last several years longer than a brand-new implant. Keeping the natural tooth will often feel more normal and can be less costly over the long-term. To help with this important decision, you can get a second opinion from a periodontist.

If you are contemplating implants, make sure your dentist doing the implants will be there when you experience the probable instance of future complications. Getting implants from a dental practice that has significant dentist turnover should be a warning flag. Find out who owns the practice and how long the dentist personally working on you has been there. Dentists are often reluctant to try to fix another dentist's mistakes. Don't get stuck in a practice with revolving door dentists for implants. If you are having an "all-on-X" type procedure, it is even more important to make sure the practice has lots of experience in this procedure, carefully evaluates your health history, and tells you all the positive and negative concepts we have discussed earlier in this book.

Referrals to dental specialists do not result in income by the initially examining dentist. Therefore, if your dentist suggests a referral, you must believe there is a reason why they suggested the referral. They may not be comfortable with that procedure or know a specialist may provide a better result for you. Do not try to convince the dentist that you think they are great and you want them to do the treatment. There is always a rationale for the referral. It is irritating to have to go to a different office, but if your dentist recommends a referral, then they are likely to be looking out for your best interests by referring you to someone who may be better at that procedure.

Conclusion

I wrote this book to help readers make the right dental decisions by providing easily understood descriptions of dental procedures and associated risks and benefits. Additionally, I hope the information provided can help you avoid dental treatment leading to excessive repairs and disappointment. It is my sincere hope that this book will assist you in properly allocating your dental healthcare dollars and help you keep your teeth for a lifetime.

It has been an honor to be your advocate for better dental health. Keep smiling!

Twenty

Glossary of Dental Terms

Author's Note

The dental terms that are defined on the following pages will better your understanding of dental care services, aid in your conversations with your dentist, and help you decipher the line items on your billing statement.

A

Abscess
A localized accumulation of pus in the tooth or gums formed by tissue infection.

Abutment
A tooth or implant used to support a dental crown or dental prosthesis.

Abutment screw
A screw used to hold a fixed or removable denture onto an implant.

Access flap procedures
Surgical techniques that reflect (cut and push back) the gums to see the roots for the purpose of improving root planing, repairing bone loss, and removing teeth.

Acid etching
Using an acidic chemical to roughen the tooth enamel for bonding.

Acute periodontal abscess
A sudden, localized accumulation of pus in the gums formed by a periodontal
infection.

Adhesive
A material that assists in joining two or more surfaces.

Aerobe
An organism that requires oxygen in its environment to survive.

Aggressive periodontitis
Periodontal disease that progresses rapidly with significant bone loss.

"All-on-X" full arch denture or prosthesis
A full arch denture or prosthesis permanently attached to dental implants. The
"X" is the number of dental implants used to attach the prosthesis to the
ridge. It is a horseshoe shape that sits above the gums but does not wrap
down the sides of the gum ridge like a traditional denture. Also called Full
Arch Implant Replacement or Hybrid Denture.

Alveolar bone
The bone that forms the sockets of the teeth and supports the teeth.

Alveoloplasty
Surgical procedure for smoothing out the jawbone, often in preparation for a
dental prosthesis.

Amalgam
A mercury and metal alloy mixture used in direct dental restorations.

Amalgam overhang

Excess filling material that projects beyond the dental preparation margins. This can trap both plaque and food leading to increased gum disease.

Anaerobe
A microorganism that can only grow in an area where there is partial or complete absence of oxygen.

Anterior
Towards the front of the mouth. Front teeth from canine to canine are anterior teeth.

Anterior tooth
A front tooth. Includes the front teeth from canine to canine.

Antibiotic therapy
Disease treatment by the local antibiotics (placed next to the tooth) or systemic antibiotics (treats whole body, such as with a pill or venous injection).

Antibody
A substance that is created by the blood system as a reaction to the presence of an antigen.

Anti-calculus agents
Compounds that inhibit or limit the formation of calculus.

Antigen
A protein that causes the formation of antibodies when introduced into a body.

Apex
The tip end of the root of the tooth.

Apical
Towards the root tip. Down the tooth away from the crown.

Apically positioned flap

The surgical sliding of gum tissue away from the bone and roots of the teeth and repositioning the tissue towards the tip of the roots to reduce pocket depths.

Apicoectomy
Surgically removing the tip of the root end of a tooth.

Arch
Either an upper or lower jaw.

Attached gingiva
Firm gum tissue that is attached to the bone by collagen fibers.

Attachment apparatus
The jawbone, periodontal ligament, and cementum attached to the tooth.

Attachment loss
A loss of ideal amounts of tissues supporting the tooth.

B

Bacterial plaque biofilm
A complex ecosystem of microbial organisms that adheres to teeth and causes inflammation if not removed.

Bass toothbrushing method
A method of toothbrushing where the toothbrush bristles are placed at a 45-degree angle to the tooth, pointed toward the gums. A wiggling motion is used to brush the bristles under the gums and between the teeth.

Benign
Non-cancerous state of an illness or growth.

Bicuspid

The teeth right behind the canines with two cusps forming the chewing surface.

Bilateral
Similarly affecting both the left and right sides of the mouth.

Biocompatibility
Acceptable to living tissues.

Biologic width
The minimum natural healthy space needed between the bottom of the periodontal pocket space and the bone. This is usually two millimeters to three millimeters. A reddened disease process is usually created if the edge of a filling or crown gets closer to the bone than the biologic width.

Biopsy
Tissue is removed for microscopic evaluation.

Bite guard
A dental appliance that is fitted over the dental arch to distribute forces evenly on the entire arch rather than on one or two teeth.

Bitewing x-ray (radiograph)
An x-ray used to look for cavities between a few teeth on one film.

Bleeding on probing
Bleeding of the gums while measuring periodontal pockets or feeling for calculus under the gums (indicates ulcers under the gums and periodontal disease).

Bone loss
A decrease in the bone levels supporting the teeth.

Bridge

A bridge is a single piece with one or more cemented crowns at each end and a fake tooth or teeth replacing the missing teeth. See diagrams for bridge below:

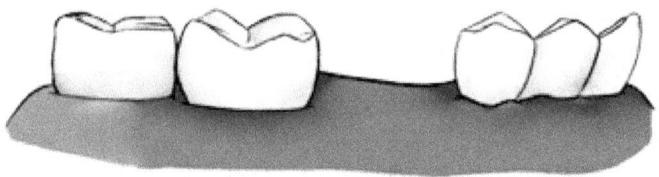

Figure 20.1. Missing lower tooth.

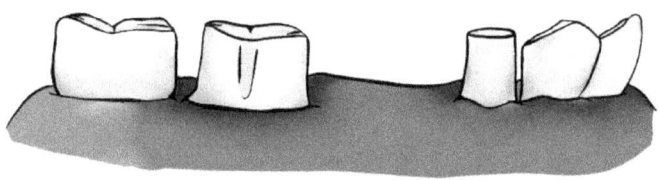

Figure 20.2. Teeth prepared (trimmed down for bridge).

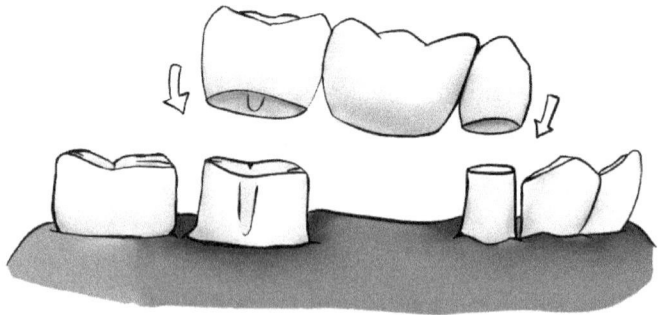

Figure 20.3. Bridge slid onto and cemented over prepared teeth.

Bruxism
The clenching or grinding of the teeth. Often done unconsciously during sleep.

Buccal
The tooth surface toward the lips or cheek.

C

Calculus
A solid mixture adhering to the teeth composed of calcium carbonate, calcium phosphate, magnesium phosphate, bacteria, dead skin cells, and other components from saliva. Calculus almost always contains live bacteria.

Cavity
Tooth decay usually caused by bacteria.

CBCT
A CBCT is an x-ray machine that takes many two-dimensional images that are reformatted to give a three-dimensional image. A CBCT image is particularly valuable for implant placement and other dental uses. Some radiation occurs with a CBCT scan, but it is important to put this into scientific perspective. Radiation damage is cumulative and particularly dangerous to children. Normal background radiation is around 7 microsieverts per day. Yearly radiation is a little under 3000 microsieverts. A plane flight from California to New York exposes you to around 500 microsieverts. A medical CT scan can range from 1000 to over 6000 microsieverts. A dental CBCT scan creates much less radiation than a full-body medical CT scan since newer dental CBCT scanners can limit the field of view to just where the dentist needs to evaluate (like where an implant is to be placed). It is reasonable to ask the dentist to limit the field of view to just the area of concern, not the entire skull. This can sometimes reduce the CBCT microsieverts of radiation to less than 100.

Cementoenamel junction

The edge where the enamel of the crown and the cementum of the root of the tooth meet. The area above the junction is the crown of the tooth; the area below the junction is the root of the tooth.

Cementum
A specialized connective tissue that covers the root of the tooth. Cementum allows for the attachment of the periodontal ligament to the root. The periodontal ligament stretches from the cementum to the jawbone.

Chemotaxis
The movement of white blood cells drawn toward an area of tissue trauma, bacteria or other microorganisms.

Chronic periodontal abscess
An abscess involving the gums and bone due to periodontal disease. Chronic implies it is long-lasting, unlike an acute periodontal abscess.

Chronic periodontitis
Periodontal disease with a long, slow course, often with bursts of episodes of tissue and bone loss. This is the most common form of periodontitis and causes the most tooth loss by adults.

Clenching
Intermittent biting down on your teeth with excess vertical pressure.

Clinical attachment loss (CAL)
A measurement of the distance from the tooth cementoenamel junction to the deepest depth of the periodontal pocket. This measurement is important because bone attachment can be lost down the tooth while keeping the same periodontal pocket depth. Without this measurement of CAL, people could incorrectly assume the disease is stable because the periodontal pocket can stay the same depth while there is loss of bone attachment to the tooth.

Combination abscess

An abscess of both the periodontal (gum) and root tip tissues, which may need both periodontal and root canal therapy or extraction of the tooth.

Compliance by the patient
The accurate completion of the doctor's prescribed course of treatment.

Composite
A tooth-colored filling material.

Comprehensive oral exam
A complete evaluation and documenting the status of the teeth and gums. Must include a periodontal diagnosis and probing measurements on all teeth.

Cover screw
A screw that is placed on top of a dental implant to protect the hole in the center of the implant from ingrowth of tissue while the implant heals to the bone.

Crepitus
Short, dry, distinctive sounds. It refers to unhealthy sounds made by the jaw joint (TMJ) when opening and closing.

Crown
The exposed portion of the tooth covered by enamel or its artificial dental replacement.

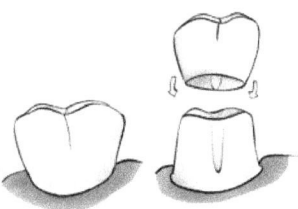

Figure 20.4. Original undisturbed tooth (left)
and prepared tooth and crown. (right)

Crown lengthening
A surgical procedure exposing more tooth for aesthetic or therapeutic reasons.

CT scan
A type of x-ray that allows three dimensional analysis of the jaws. This type of x-ray can be invaluable for implants, orthodontics, and root canals. CT scans expose the patient to much more radiation than traditional dental x-rays and some researchers are concerned that overuse of CT scans will lead to an increase in cancer deaths.

Cusp
The large bumps on the biting surfaces of back teeth. Molars can have four or five cusps.

D

Decay
Decomposing of tooth structure.

Deciduous teeth
The normal twenty primary or baby teeth.

Dental implant
A device placed within the bone to hold an artificial tooth or to support a dental appliance.

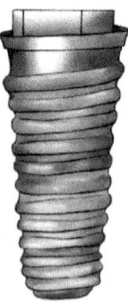

Figure 20.5. Dental implant (also called implant fixture or implant body).

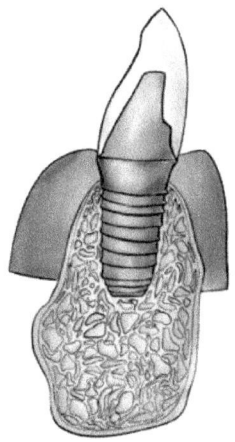

*Figure 20.6. Cross section of a crown on an abutment
attached to a dental implant in the jawbone.*

Dental plaque biofilm
Bacteria and other microbes accumulating on the teeth. A biofilm is sticky and
must be scraped or brushed off since rinsing will not remove it.

Dental prophylaxis
A scaling and polishing procedure which removes plaque and stain.

Dental prosthesis
An artificial replacement of a tooth or teeth.

Dentin
The central solid body of the tooth that is covered by enamel and cementum.
Contains the nerves and blood supply.

Dentin sensitivity
The uncomfortable response of tooth dentin to temperature, sweets, fluids,
and scraping.

Dentinal hypersensitivity

Extreme dentin and tooth sensitivity after the root dentin is uncovered due to trauma, disease, or a dental procedure.

Dentinal tubules
There are tiny tubes in the root dentin that traverse horizontally from the central blood and nerve supply to the edges of the tooth root. These tubules contain nerves that can be sensitive to temperature, sweets, trauma, and liquids if the root surface is exposed.

Denture
An artificial substitute for teeth and gums.

Diagnostic cast
Plaster model of teeth used for planning dental treatment.

Direct pulp cap
A dental procedure where the exposed nerve or pulp is covered by a medication or material.

Distal
The surface of the tooth (not the cheek or tongue side) toward the back of the mouth and more distant from the midline of the face.

Dry socket
A painful inflammation of the tooth socket following extraction due to infection or loss of the blood clot.

E

Early-onset periodontitis
Periodontal disease affecting children and teenagers.

Edentulous
Without any teeth.

Embrasure

The space that is created below the contact areas of the adjacent touching teeth.

Endodontic abscess
An abscess involving the dental pulp and nerves.

Endodontist
A dentist with two to three extra years of special training who limits their practice to root canal treatment.

Endotoxin
Microscopic components released by dead bacteria that can produce an immunological response by the body.

Epithelium
The thin layer of skin tissue covering our bodies.

Excision
The surgical removal of soft tissue or bone.

Exostosis
Heavy overgrowth of bone.

Extraction
The removal of a tooth or parts of a tooth.

F

Failing implant
A dental implant with significant and increasing infection and bone loss.

Filling
The restoration of removed or lost tooth structure.

Food impaction areas

Areas between teeth where food becomes lodged. These areas are often caused by loose or open contacts between teeth or uneven edges between teeth or tooth cusps (plunger cusps) from the opposing arch hitting directly into the space where food becomes impacted.

Fremitus
Excessive movement of a tooth during normal and abnormal function.

Frenum
The tissue composed of a narrow band of fibers that connect parts of the mouth together (gums to lips, cheek and tongue).

Full arch implant replacement
A full arch denture or prosthesis permanently attached to dental implants. Also called an "all-on-X" prosthesis. The "X" is the number of dental implants used to attach the prosthesis to the ridge. It is a horseshoe shape that sits above the gums but does not wrap down the sides of the gum ridge like a traditional denture. Also called a hybrid denture.

Full denture
A removable acrylic and plastic or ceramic tooth substitute for all the natural teeth and gums in one arch.

Full mouth debridement
The full mouth removal of plaque and calculus to see the teeth and gums to enable an evaluation.

Furcation
The region of a tooth where the main root (trunk) divides into two or more smaller roots.

G

Gingiva
The tough tissue that immediately surrounds the teeth. The visible part of the periodontal tissues next to the teeth.

Gingival abscess
A periodontal abscess in the surface tissues around the tooth. It is usually caused by food like a popcorn husk.

Gingival crevicular fluid
A fluid that leaks out of the space between the gums and teeth (gingival sulcus or pocket). Local gum infection can increase the flow of this fluid.

Gingival curettage
Removing the lining of tissue in the periodontal pocket. Its value has been called into question in recent decades.

Gingival enlargement
An abnormal increase in the size of the gingiva. Often caused by certain drugs.

Gingival margin
The visible edge of the gums next to the teeth.

Gingival recession
The migration of the gums exposing more tooth due to disease or trauma.

Gingivectomy
The surgical removal of unsupported gum tissue, creating a new level of the gum tissue. This can reduce periodontal pocket depth.

Gingivitis
Inflammation of the gum tissues.

Gingivoplasty
The surgical smoothing of the gum tissue.

Gram-negative cell wall
A type of cell wall structure of a bacteria. Gram-negative can indicate more aggressive bacteria.

Gram-positive cell wall

A type of cell wall structure of a bacteria. Gram-positive can indicate less aggressive bacteria.

Guided tissue regeneration

Controlling the regrowth of specific types of cells.

H

Healing abutment

An implant abutment that screws into the implant fixture and sticks through the gums to allow the tissue to heal in a circle around it.

Horizontal bone loss

Periodontal bone loss where the crest of the bone between teeth is reduced but remains level.

Hybrid denture

A full arch denture or prosthesis permanently attached to dental implants. Also called an "all-on-X" prosthesis. The "X" is the number of dental implants used to attach the prosthesis to the ridge. It is a horseshoe shape that sits above the gums but does not wrap down the sides of the gum ridge like a traditional denture. Also called full-arch implant rehabilitation.

Hydrodynamic causes of dentinal sensitivity

Tooth sensitivity can be due to the movement of fluids in the dentinal tubules. This fluid movement over the nerves in the tubules in the dentin can cause pain.

Hyperplasia

An enlargement of the gum tissue by increase of the number of gum cells.

I

Immediate denture

A denture (usually temporary) placed immediately after the extractions of teeth.

Immediate loading
Placement of the crown or other dental restoration at the same time of the implant placement surgery.

Immune system
The system of cells in the body that respond to infection and trauma.

Immunoglobulin
Proteins your body makes that act as antibodies and fight against infections. Types of immunoglobulins are IgA, IgD, IgE, IgG, and IgM.

Impacted tooth
A tooth blocked from erupting. Usually, another tooth is in the way.

Implant abutment
The part of an implant that sticks through the gums and is designed to hold a dental crown or appliance. Abutments can be used for cement retention, screw retention, or an O-ring attachment retention.

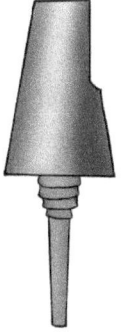

Figure 20.7. Implant abutment.

Implant biologic width

The height of the epithelium (gum skin) plus the connective tissue above the bone next to a dental implant. This is slightly different than biologic width against a natural tooth.

Implant fixture (implant body)

The part of a dental implant that replaces a tooth root.

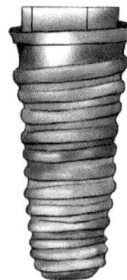

Figure 20.8. Dental implant (also called implant fixture or implant body).

Incisal

The biting surface of a front tooth.

Incisional periodontal surgery

Periodontal flap surgery. The periodontal surgery where the gum tissue is pushed back to reveal and treat the tooth roots and bone.

Indirect pulp cap

A medicament or other material is placed over a nearly exposed pulp.

Informed consent

Written and/or verbal explanation of the risks and expectations of a particular treatment anticipated for a patient before treatment is rendered. This explanation is provided to allow the patient to intelligently accept or reject treatment.

Informed refusal
A written or verbal patient refusal to proceed with treatment after the risks of the treatment versus no treatment have been explained.

Inlay
A laboratory created dental restoration that does not include the tooth cusps.

Interdental brushes
Small brushes used to clean between the teeth, one space at a time.

Interim denture
A dental prosthesis designed for use over a limited amount of time. A more permanent denture will be fabricated after the tissues have healed and/or adequate evaluation has occurred during this initial amount of time.

Interproximal
The surfaces between the teeth where mesial surface of a tooth touches the distal surface of an adjacent tooth.

Intraoral
The area inside the mouth.

Intravenous sedation
A method to medically induce a state of reduced consciousness while the patient's breathing, reflexes, and the ability to respond to stimuli are maintained. This state is achieved by administering drugs into the bloodstream in a titrated amount to match the patient's tolerance.

Irrigation

Rinsing or flushing material from the periodontal pocket, a root canal, or a wound.

Intaglio surface
The underside of a denture or removable partial. The surface that is placed in contact with the gum tissue over the jawbone.

J

Jaw
People all have two jaws. The upper jaw (maxilla) is fused and part of the bones of the skull. The other jaw is the lower (mandible) which is held to the skull via muscles and ligaments. Since the lower jaw (mandible) is not fused to the skull, it can move in many directions to allow speech and eating, etc.

Jumping distance
The cross section of an extracted tooth is rarely perfectly round, and most implants are perfectly round. If an implant is placed in a tooth socket immediately upon extraction, a gap can exist between the implant surface and part of the inner aspect of the tooth socket wall. If this gap is small, your body can fill it in with bone and attach to the implant. This small space is called the jumping distance.

Junctional epithelium
The band of skin cells that attaches to and surround the tooth. They create a tight seal to the tooth.

L

Lesion
An area of trauma, disease, or wound.

Limited oral evaluation
An exam that is focused on specific problem the patient has that is most bothersome.

Lingual

The surface of the tooth facing the tongue.

Loading
The placement of dental restorations on dental implants. These restorations are possibly in contact with the teeth on the opposite arch.

Local anesthesia
An injection of anesthetic that creates a loss of sensation over an area of tissue. The patient is awake, but the tissues are numb.

Localized aggressive periodontitis
A fast moving, destructive periodontal disease often associated with young people.

M

Malocclusion
A deviation in the ideal relationships between the teeth and possibly between the upper and lower arches.

Mandible
The lower jaw.

Maryland bridge
A glued-on bridge done with no or nearly no trimming down of the teeth. This helps keep valuable tooth structure but can have a weaker attachment than a traditional fixed bridge.

Materia alba
A loosely attached mix of bacteria, pieces of dead cells, and food around the teeth. Materia alba can be rinsed away, unlike dental plaque which sticks solidly to teeth.

Maxilla
The upper arch that is solidly attached to the skull.

Mesial
The surface of the tooth toward the midline (front center) of the mouth.

Microbial succession
As plaque ages undisturbed, the types of bacteria in dental plaque change in composition towards more damaging, oxygen-intolerant species of bacteria. This is called microbial succession.

Miller Index (for Tooth Mobility)
A way to quantify tooth mobility. Dental instrument handles are used to push on a tooth from the tongue side towards the cheek side and back. The tooth is rated on a scale of 0 to 3, with 3 being most mobile. A measurement of tooth mobility is recorded in the dental chart.

Molar
The three large back teeth in each corner of the mouth. Includes the wisdom teeth.

Mouth breathing
Breathing in and out through your mouth, rather than through your nose. This can dry out and irritate the gum tissues.

Mucous membrane
The moist layer of skin cells lining the mouth.

N

Necrotizing ulcerative gingivitis (NUG)
An inflammation and infection of the gums characterized by a depression of dead gum tissue between the teeth. Usually produces a bad smell. Commonly seen occurring in people under stress, often associated with students during final exams.

Necrotizing ulcerative periodontitis (NUP)

An inflammation and infection of the gums characterized by dead gum tissue between the teeth and simultaneously destroying bone in addition to the soft gum tissue. Usually produces a bad smell.

Nightguard An acrylic appliance that is worn to minimize damage to the teeth from excessive clenching or grinding. The nightguard distributes the pressures on the entire arch so one or two teeth do not receive all the forces of the clenching.

Nitrous oxide
Also called laughing gas. A titrated mixture of gases that are inhaled to relax the patient. The effect wears off in only a few minutes once the patient starts breathing oxygen or normal room air.

Non-submerged implant protocol
The dental implant is placed leaving the healing abutment protruding through the gum tissue. This eliminates needing a second surgery to uncover the implant. This sounds great, but it is not ideal in circumstances where the patient has some biologic compromises.

Nonsurgical periodontal therapy
Scaling and root planing procedures and occasional antimicrobial agents to try to control periodontitis.

O

Obligate anaerobe
A microorganism that cannot survive in an environment full of oxygen. For example, the surface of the teeth exposed in the mouth would be a tough environment for an obligate anaerobe. Obligate anaerobes do well deep under the gums away from the air in your mouth.

Occlusal
The horizontal surface of a back tooth used for chewing.

Occlusion

A description of how the chewing surfaces of the teeth meet together with the teeth of the opposing arch.

Operculum
A piece of tissue lying over a partially erupted tooth. This is often seen with partially erupted wisdom teeth. Pericoronitis is the infection that can occur under the operculum.

Oral
Beyond the lips inside the mouth.

Oral prophylaxis
The cleaning of the teeth.

Orthodontist
A specialist trained for two to three years beyond dental school in the treatment of the alignment of the teeth and jaws.

Osseointegration
The healed attachment of bone tissue to dental implants.

Osseous defects
Bone loss adjacent to teeth usually resulting from periodontal disease.

Osseous surgery
Surgical treatment to reduce or eliminate jawbone deformities created by bone destruction seen in periodontitis. The objective is to create an area that is easier to clean for the patient and dental hygienist. This usually means making periodontal pockets shallower.

Ostectomy
The surgical removal of bone or a piece of bone.

Osteoplasty
A surgical procedure to change the local shape of the jawbone.

Over-contoured crowns

Crowns made by a laboratory where the natural tooth shape was not replicated, and a crown edge or extra crown material protrudes from the ideal shape. This can trap bacterial plaque and food causing periodontal disease.

Over-contoured filling

A dental filling that protrudes beyond the normal shape of a tooth. This can trap bacterial plaque and food causing periodontal disease.

Overdenture

A removable denture supported by retained tooth roots or dental implants.

P

Palate

The roof of the mouth above the tongue.

Panoramic x-ray

An x-ray of the entire jaw, teeth, and adjacent areas of tissue and bone. It is taken with a rotating x-ray head from outside of the mouth, without placing film inside the mouth. It provides excellent information for some things, but it is usually not as detailed as periapical or bitewing x-rays.

Papillae

A natural bump of gum tissue filling the spaces between teeth.

Parafunctional activity

Bruxism, grinding, or clenching jaw movements that are not normal and not used during eating.

Partial denture

A dental device that replaces missing teeth. It can be removable (the patient can take it out to clean it) or fixed (permanently glued or screwed on).

Periapical
Around or at the root tip.

Periapical abscess
An infection or inflammation of the tissues around the root tip.

Periapical x-ray
An x-ray (radiograph) made by exposing film or a digital sensor that was placed
in the mouth next to the teeth. It is used for evaluating the health of the
tooth root tips and the shape and position of roots.

Pericoronitis
Infection or inflammation of the tissue around and over a partially erupted
tooth, especially seen on wisdom teeth.

Peri-implant disease
Disease in the tissues around a dental implant.

Peri-implant mucositis
Inflammation of the gum tissue around a dental implant and abutment that
can be controlled with dental hygiene treatment.

Peri-implantitis
Infection and Inflammation of the gum tissue and bone around a dental
implant and abutment.

Periodic oral evaluation
Dental evaluation used to compare the current status to the previous health or
disease status.

Periodontal
The tissues surrounding the teeth.

Periodontal abscess
A localized infection of the gum tissues around the teeth with pus and swelling.

Periodontal bone loss
The loss of bone supporting the teeth bone due to periodontal disease.

Periodontal disease
Any one of many different infectious diseases and types of inflammatory processes affecting the gums and tissues supporting the teeth.

Periodontal dressing
A temporary dressing placed over the gum tissues after periodontal surgery to minimize food impaction and minimize tissue mobility.

Periodontal flap surgery
Making a surgical incision and pushing back the gum tissue to clean the teeth and treat periodontal disease.

Periodontal ligament
The set of specialized cells attaching a tooth root to the jawbone. It allows for slight tooth movement and responds to pressure.

Periodontal maintenance
Dental hygiene therapy to help control and prevent periodontal disease.

Periodontal plastic surgery
The surgical treatment of the periodontium for cosmetic or support purposes.
Periodontal pocket
A space between the teeth and gums that has been deepened by disease.

Periodontal surgery
Surgery on the gums next to the teeth.

Periodontics
The study of the diagnosis and treatment of diseases affecting the gums and bone around teeth.

Periodontist
A dentist who went to an additional three years after dental school to specialize in gum disease and dental implants.

Periodontitis
Inflammation and disease resulting in loss of bone supporting the teeth.

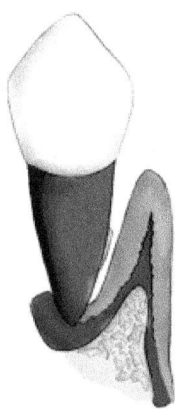

Figure 20.9. Periodontal disease has destroyed all gum and bone support on this tooth.

Periodontium
The set of specialized cells and tissues that support the teeth.

Permanent teeth
The adult set of teeth. Normally consisting of thirty-two teeth, but many adults never get all four of their wisdom teeth.

Physiologic mobility
The minor and normal movement of the teeth when pressed upon.

Plaque
The sticky material that accumulates on teeth. Plaque mostly consists of bacteria and the products the bacteria make.

Pocket reduction surgery
The use of periodontal surgery to reduce the depth of an existing periodontal pocket to make it less conducive for destructive bacteria to live in and easier for the patient and hygienist to clean.

Polishing
The use of polishing agents in a rotating rubber cup to remove stains and plaque from the teeth.

Pontic
The fake tooth between the teeth a fixed partial denture (bridge) is cemented to.

Post
A toothpick-shaped piece of material cemented in a root canal to help support a crown.

Posterior
The back teeth. The teeth behind the canines.

Pregnancy tumor
A localized swelling of easily bleeding gum tissue, magnified by pregnancy hormonal changes. Occasionally pregnancy tumors go away after the baby is born, but they often require removal by surgery.

Premolar
In adults, the two teeth directly behind the canines. Older terminology called them bicuspids.

Probing measurements
Records of the depth of sulcus or periodontal pockets in millimeters.

Prognosis
The normally expected course of a disease.

Prophylaxis
The cleaning and polishing procedures done to help control dental diseases.

Pulp
The nerve and blood supply in the center of the tooth.

Pulpotomy
Surgically removing part of the pulp.

Purulence
Pus or exudate consisting of blood serum and cells.

Q

Quadrant
One of four equally-divided sections of the mouth. For instance, the upper
right quadrant is the area of the maxilla on the patient's right side from
the midline back.

R

Rapidly progressing periodontitis
Periodontitis that causes severe, rapid gum tissue inflammation and periodontal bone loss.

Rebase
Replacing the base material of a denture and keeping the original denture
teeth.

Recession
A reduced level of the tissue margin of the gums exposing the root.

Recurrent periodontitis
Periodontal disease that returns after periodontal treatment.

Reevaluation
A review of progress after an initial evaluation or treatment.

Refractory periodontitis
Periodontal disease that does not come under control by treatment that normally controls the disease.

Reline
Placing a new layer of material on the tissue side of the denture.

Risk factors
A behavior or exposure that increases the risk of getting a disease.

Root
The portion of the tooth holding the tooth in the jawbone. The root is normally hidden from view by the gums.

Root canal
The portion of the pulp chamber that extends down the center of the root or roots of the tooth. It's removal and replacement is also called a root canal.

Root canal treatment
The blood vessels and nerve of the tooth is removed from the canal in the center of the root and replaced with a rubber-like material cemented in place.

Root caries
Decay occurring on the root.

Root planing
A procedure that scrapes away bacteria, calculus, and contaminated root surface.

Rubber tip stimulators
A cone-shaped piece of rubber on a toothbrush-type handle used to rub away bacteria on the tooth roots.

S

Scaling
The removal of bacteria and calculus from the teeth by use of dental instruments.

Silver diamine fluoride
A topical solution that can stop around 80% of cavities from getting worse. This is a particularly effective and simple treatment for nursing home residents and at risk children.

Subgingival
Under the gums.

Subgingival calculus
Calculus on the tooth below the gums.

Subgingival irrigation
The flushing of liquid beneath the gum line.

Subgingival plaque biofilm
Plaque that is located below the gums in the sulcus or periodontal pocket.

Submerged protocol
A technique where the dental implant is placed in the bone and then covered fully by the gum tissue which is sutured over it. After healing, the implant is exposed by a second surgery and an implant abutment is placed to allow the gums to heal around the abutment. This implant technique requires two surgical procedures. The first surgery places the implant in bone. The second surgery is done three to six months later to uncover the implant and place the implant abutment.

Sulcus
The normal shallow space between the gums and the tooth where popcorn husks or hulls can get stuck. When a sulcus gets deeper due to gum disease or gum enlargement, the space is called a periodontal pocket.

Suppuration

The discharge of pus.

Supragingival calculus
Calculus on the teeth visible above the gums.

Suture
A stitch used to repair an injury or surgically opened area.

T

Tartar
Another term for dental calculus.

Temporomandibular disorder (TMD)
A disorder associated with the temporomandibular joints (TMJ).

Temporary denture
An artificial substitute for teeth and gums that is meant for short term use to facilitate healing changes.

Titanium
A biocompatible metal that is the most common material used for dental implants.

Tooth mobility
How much a tooth wiggles under function or by measuring movement side to side. More mobility than normal often indicates pathology – bone loss or heavy function.

Tooth root proximity
How close roots are to each other.

Tooth wear
Wearing down teeth surfaces due to the friction of teeth rubbing on each other.

Torus

A bump of bone often seen in the center of the palate or the sides of the jaw-bones. It is often benign.

Traumatic occlusion
The way teeth meet with the opposing arch that causes injury to the TMJ, muscles, or other teeth.

Trismus
A spasm of the jaw muscles that can cause pain and difficulty in opening the mouth.

U

Ultrasonic instrumentation
A dental device that uses high-frequency vibrations to remove calculus, plaque, and stain. Often called a Cavitron®, ultrasonic scaler, or piezo scaler.

Unerupted
A tooth that has not erupted through the gum tissue into the mouth.

V

Vertical bone loss
In vertical bone loss, more bone has been destroyed on the side of one tooth compared to the bone on the nearest side of the adjacent tooth.

X

Xerostomia
Dry mouth. Xerostomia is commonly caused by hundreds of different pre-scribed medications. Dry mouth can also be caused by medical conditions affecting the salivary glands.

About the Author

Dr. Mark Morgan graduated magna cum laude with Alpha Sigma Nu honors from Santa Clara University. He received his doctorate from UCLA School of Dentistry with Omicron Kappa Upsilon honors and was the recipient of the American Academy of Periodontology annual student award. He completed a specialist residency in periodontology at the University of California, San Francisco. He is also a Diplomate of the American Sleep and Breathing Academy. He received a Master of Business Administration degree from the University of Texas at Austin.

Dr. Morgan is a life member of the American Dental Association. He has had a varied career working as a general dentist, periodontist, emergency clinic dentist, implantologist, free clinic volunteer, and a volunteer providing care in mobile buses to migrant farm workers. He has worked for a multi-location corporate practice and has owned his own offices employing multiple dentists and hygienists. He spent several years teaching dental students and dental hygiene students as a clinical instructor and assistant professor. Dr. Morgan served as a clinical tester for localized antibiotic therapy in the FDA approval process.

Dr. Morgan's background has led him to a broad understanding of dentistry and the difficulty patients face getting quality, cost-effective dental treatment.

www.ingramcontent.com/pod-product-compliance
Lightning Source LLC
Chambersburg PA
CBHW060139130626
46556CB00006B/2411